ORTHOPAEDIC MRI

A Teaching File Approach

ORTHOPAEDIC MRI

A Teaching File Approach

JOHN H. BISESE, M.D.

Georgia Baptist Medical Center
Atlanta Magnetic Imaging
(A Division of Health Images, Inc.)
Atlanta, Georgia

McGRAW-HILL INFORMATION SERVICES COMPANY
Health Professions Division

New York   St. Louis   San Francisco   Colorado Springs   Auckland
Bogotá   Caracas   Hamburg   Lisbon   London   Madrid   Mexico   Milan   Montreal
New Delhi   Paris   San Juan   São Paulo   Singapore   Sydney   Tokyo   Toronto

ORTHOPAEDIC MRI: A TEACHING FILE APPROACH

234567890 HDHD 99876543210

ISBN 0-07-005404-5

This book was set in Melior by Compset.

The editors were Sally J. Barhydt and Mariapaz Ramos-Englis.

The production supervisor was Annette Mayeski.

The text and cover were designed and the project
was supervised by M 'N O Production Services, Inc.

Arcata Graphics/Halliday was the printer and binder.

Library of Congress Cataloging-in-Publication Data

Bisese, John H.
    Orthopaedic MRI : a teaching file approach / John H. Bisese.
        p.   cm.
    Includes bibliographical references.
    ISBN 0-07-005404-5
    1. Orthopedics—Diagnosis—Atlases.   2. Magnetic
resonance imaging—Atlases.   I. Title.
    [DNLM: 1. Magnetic Resonance Imaging—
atlases.   2. Orthopedics—atlases.   WE 17 B621o]
RD734.5.M33B57   1990
617.3—dc20
DNLM/DLC
for Library of Congress   89-13043
                                                          CIP

To my darling bride, Ann,
and our boys, Danny and Scott

CONTENTS

ACKNOWLEDGMENTS

I would like to express my thanks to the following people: The patients, staff, and medical residents of Georgia Baptist Medical Center; Health Images, Inc., and its President and Chairman/Chief Executive Officer, Robert D. Carl III; Kathy deLacy and her staff at Atlanta Magnetic Imaging-South; Donna Sheffield and her staff at Atlanta Magnetic Imaging; Pamela Pittard and her staff at Athens Magnetic Imaging, Ltd.; and Craig Allen and his staff at Central PA Magnetic Imaging, Ltd.

Also thanks to Maryland Magnetic Imaging; Pasadena Magnetic Imaging, Ltd.; Philadelphia Magnetic Imaging, Ltd.; and Northeastern Magnetic Imaging, Ltd.

Special appreciation to Sandra Brum and Dorrine Moore, Marketing Division, and Perry Polsinelli and Michael Scott, Engineering Division, Health Images, Inc.

A special thanks to Valerie, John, Beth, Sylvia, Kristi, Gina, Christy, Jerri, John C., Robin, Ann, Bill, Len, and Debbie.

PREFACE

In the summer of 1985 we began interpreting magnetic resonance studies performed at a privately owned magnet based in the northern part of metropolitan Atlanta. This was the first clinically operational magnet in the area and offered us a unique opportunity to gain early and extensive clinical experience with MRI. Within a year, we also began to interpret studies performed on a magnet based in downtown Atlanta. As our experience grew, the number of interesting cases accumulated rapidly. We subsequently published a compilation of 250 of what we considered to be the most effective teaching cases in MRI: A TEACHING FILE APPROACH (McGraw-Hill, 1988). Based on our success with that book, we were encouraged to move from the general to the specific.

This new volume focuses on one of the significant subsets of cases, the orthopaedic realm, which we have encountered as routine clinical problems. Orthopaedic surgeons are naturally interested in the lumbar and cervical spine applications. In addition, a significant number of knee and shoulder cases as well as cases of other extremity masses resulting from trauma and tumor present excellent subjects for MRI investigation. Such cases may be equally useful for neurologists and neurosurgeons and residents in these specialties.

The format of ORTHOPAEDIC MRI follows that of the previous book. The emphasis in these 275 representative cases is on the MR appearance of the pathology. Three or four illustrations are shown for each case, and the question, "What does it look like?" is addressed throughout.

It should be noted that the cases presented here were all seen in a busy clinical hospital and in an outpatient community setting and therefore represent commonly encountered problems. It is our intent in this atlas to provide a convenient and practical reference source for orthopaedic MR imaging that will prove of value to the orthopaedic surgeon and radiologist alike and their residents.

John H. Bisese, M.D.

ORTHOPAEDIC MRI

A Teaching File Approach

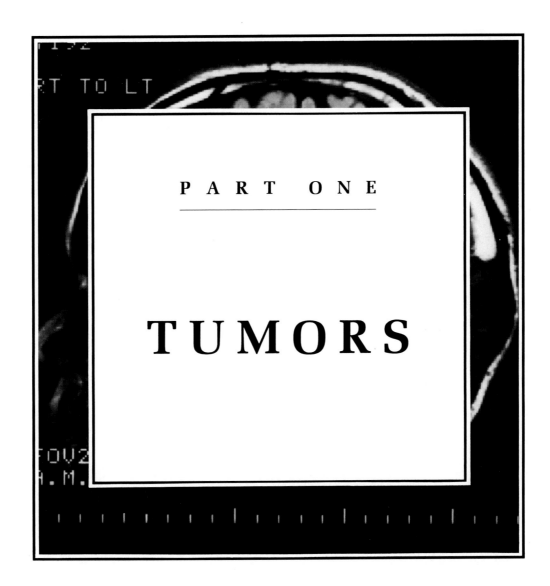

PART ONE

TUMORS

1.1 HEMANGIOMA OF THE LUMBAR VERTEBRAL BODY

These lesions should be regarded as an incidental finding. They are benign vascular malformations. They exhibit a characteristic high signal on the T1- and T2-weighted images. They can involve a small portion of the body or replace it almost entirely. The outer contour of the lesion is discrete. Figure 1 demonstrates the sagittal view of a typical hemangioma (arrow).

Figure 2 is typical of the sagittal appearance of such lesions (arrow).

Figure 3 shows the T2-weighted appearance. The differential diagnosis of such lesions can be focal fatty metamorphosis of the bone marrow. On occasion, metastases can bleed and simulate hemangiomas, but these are usually multiple and have secondary destructive signs.

Some hemangiomas can grow out into the epidural space and cause canal obstruction. However, this behavior is unusual.

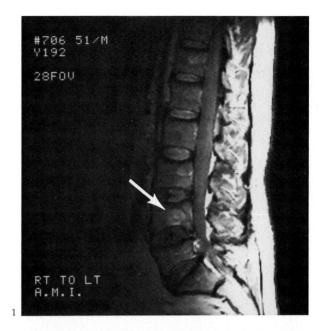

1

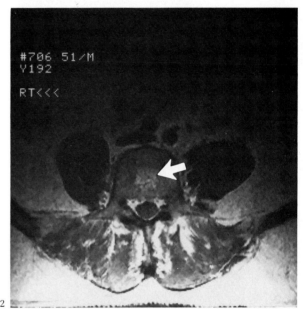

2

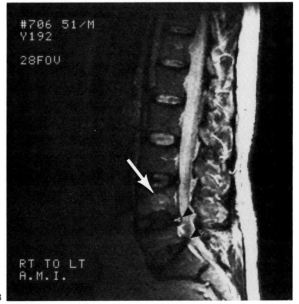

3

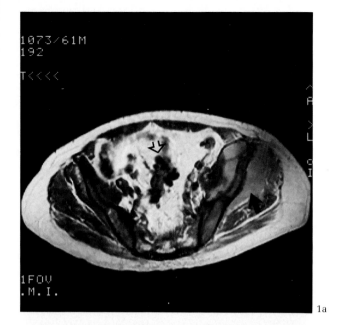

1a

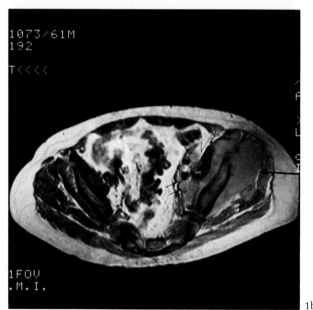

1b

1.2 RENAL METASTASIS TO PELVIS BONE

Figures 1a and 1b demonstrate large, destructive lesions to the iliac bone with a large amount of extra osseous tissue (large arrows). There is also a large amount of adenopathy to the iliac chain (small arrows).

Figure 2a is a coronal magnetic resonance imaging (MRI) cut through the pelvis, which can include some of the upper abdominal contents if the patient is small enough. This particular cut demonstrates the cause of the bone mets by showing the primary renal cell carcinoma (large arrow).

Figure 2b demonstrates the metastatic involvement in the coronal plane. Note the characteristic decrease in signal seen with the underlying metastatic change within the normally high-signal bone marrow regions. The large amount of exophytic soft tissue further supports a diagnosis of malignant cause of this bone abnormality.

Figure 3 is a plain film of the pelvis. A tiny area of cortical destruction is noted, but the changes seen here vastly underestimate the amount of full-blown bone destruction.

At this time, MRI is too slow an imaging procedure to include a whole body survey as a reasonable application. It is better to focus on a suspicious portion of the body, particularly when the plain film or even the nuclear bone scan is negative but the clinical suspicion remains high. Incidental note is made of the diverticular changes to the sigmoid colon (Figure 1, open arrow).

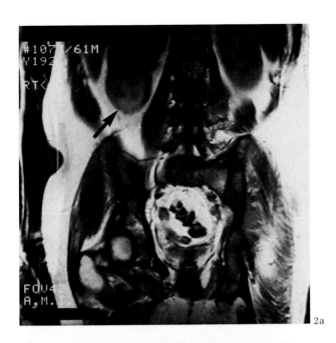

2a

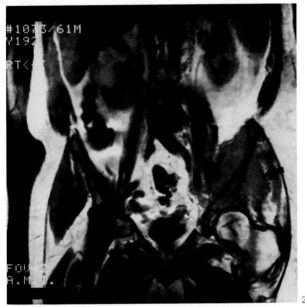

2b

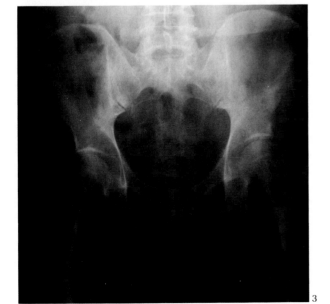

3

1.3 FIBROUS DYSPLASIA OF THE OCCIPITAL BONE

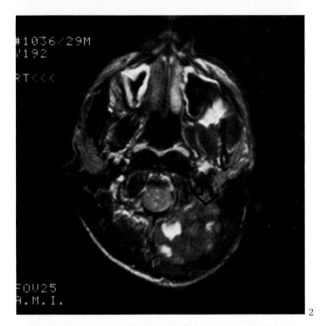

1

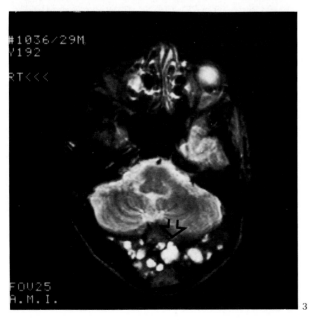

2

3

This is a dramatic example of fibrous dysplasia involving the bone of the calvaria. Figure 1 demonstrates the features of intrinsic expansion of the bone without extension into the cranial vault. However, note the extrinsic compression of the posterior fossa contents.

Figures 2 and 3 demonstrate the multiple cysts and expansion that appear to arise from the diploic spaces.

The extrinsic effect seen here helps to demonstrate that when this process affects the foraminal bones, cranial nerve paralysis can result.

1.4 ENCHONDROMA OF THE MIDTIBIAL SHAFT

A well-marginated, low-signal structure is identified on Figure 1 in the midshaft of the left tibia. There is a well-demarcated edge, and this is an intramedullary structure. It has a well-defined border and can be easily separated from the high-signal fat (see Figures 2 and 3). The axial images on Figure 3 demonstrate the nice interface between the high-signal bone marrow designated by the small arrow and the low-signal enchondroma. This lesion has the features of a benign lesion; however, some metastases identified on MRI may have the same well-marginated appearance, and clinical correlation is necessary. Also, plain films should always augment MRI studies of the extremities.

This case is through the courtesy of Dr. Robert Chiteman of Maryland Magnetic Imaging.

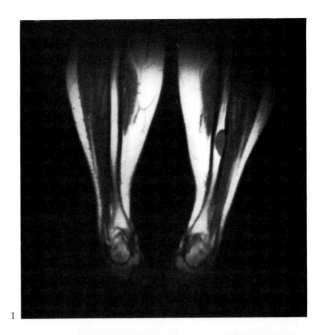

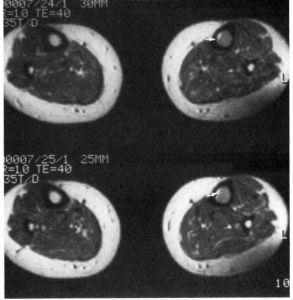

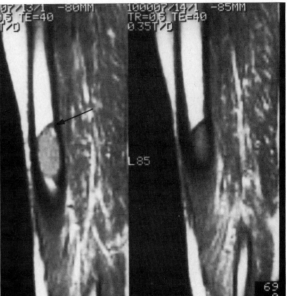

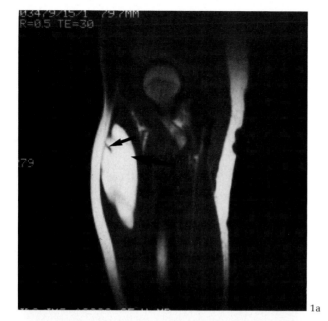

1a

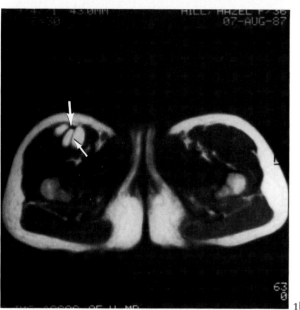

1b

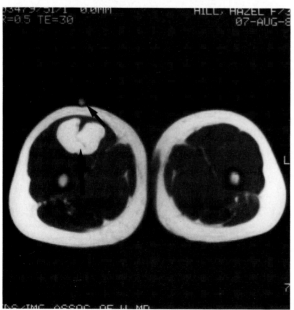

2

1.5 LIPOMA OF THE RECTUS FEMORIS

Figure 1a is a sagittal cut through the thigh. Figure 1b is an axial cut through this area. The large arrow demonstrates a mass with septation representing stretched but retained muscle fibers (small arrow). Figure 2 is a T1 proton density-weighted image, again demonstrating, in a slightly lower cut, the well-rounded, high-signal structure with some muscle traversing this structure. The small arrow indicates a small water bottle placed over the area of clinical interest. Figure 3a is a T1-weighted image, and Figures 2 and 3b are T2-weighted images through this same structure, demonstrating the isointense behavior of the material within this tumor with that of the subcutaneous tissues of the thigh (curved arrow). The differential diagnosis for a fairly well-circumscribed structure with a high signal behaving in this manner would be subacute hematoma. However, hematomas normally expand the muscle fiber from the point where they arise and do not arise in several compartments where lipomatous masses may invade and grow along the interstitial plane separating the numerous muscle bundles. A history of recent trauma and an acute appearance of a mass rather than a mass that has been present for a long time, as in this patient, would help increase the suspicion of a hematoma.

As always, all striations through the lipoma should be viewed with suspicion as possibly representing a more malignant component. The possibility of a liposarcoma should also be considered.

This case is through the courtesy of Dr. Robert Chiteman of Maryland Magnetic Imaging.

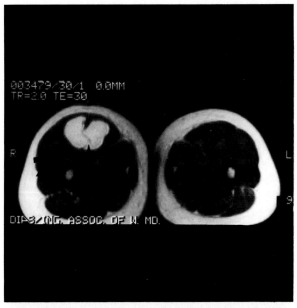

003479/30/1 0.0MM
TR=2.0 TE=30
R
L
DIAG/ING. ASSOC. OF W. MD.

3a

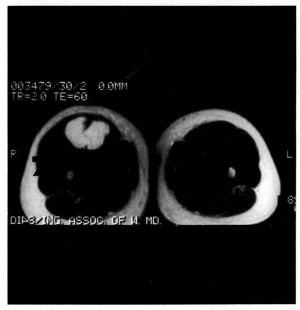

003479/30/2 0.0MM
TR=2.0 TE=60
R
L
DIAG/ING. ASSOC. OF W. MD.

3b

1.6 NONOSSIFYING FIBROMA

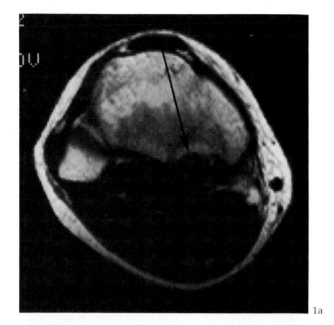

1a

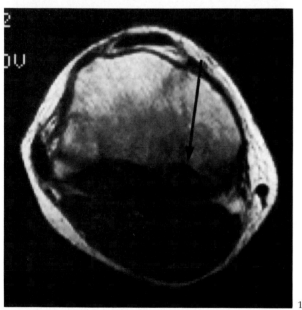

1b

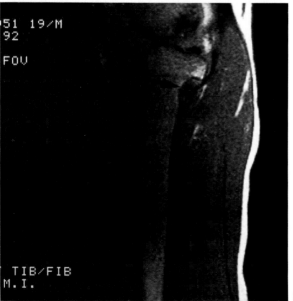

2

Incidental plain film findings in a 19-year-old male were sent for evaluation with MRI. The well-marginated, slightly sclerotic border of a structure in the posterior proximal tibial shaft is identified on the MRI scans (Figures 1a, 1b, and 2, arrows). It has a partially scalloped appearance. There is no extraosseous soft tissue mass. This appearance correlates well with that of the benign, nonossifying fibroma, which is also illustrated on a plain film (Figures 3a and 3b). The MRI scan duplicates some of the findings on the plain film but increases the physician's diagnostic ability by demonstrating the characteristics of the soft tissues. It is particularly sensitive to any extraosseous extension of a bone lesion; this can sometimes be quite helpful in determining the malignant potential of a bone lesion.

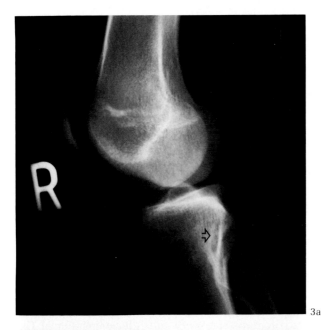

3a

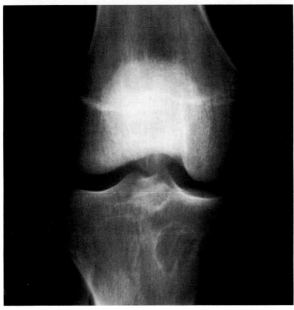

3b

11

1.7 METASTASIS TO THE FEMORAL SHAFT

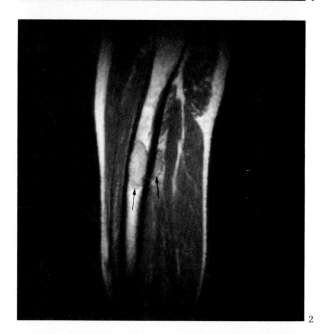

1

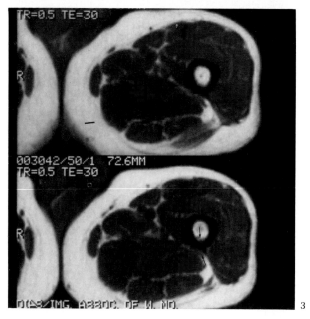

2

Coronal images of this 64-year-old female demonstrate a fairly discrete, fairly well-marginated area of decreased signal intensity in the left femoral shaft (Figure 1). The large arrow indicates the inferior aspect of the lesion, the small arrow the superior aspect. The cortex appears normal and of uniform thickness.

MRI is useful in demonstrating extraosseous extension despite the apparent integrity of the cortex. Note the soft tissue excrescence from the intramedullary process into the subcutaneous tissues surrounding the cortex (Figure 2). Small arrows demonstrate both the inferior aspect of the intramedullary process and the exophytic portion of the process.

The axial images on Figure 3 (small arrows) demonstrate abnormal soft tissue on both sides of the cortex. At first glance, this lesion appears to be fairly well circumscribed and suggests a benign process such as an enchondroma, fibrodysplasia, or even a simple bone cyst. However, with additional images, the transgression of the cortical bone is identified. Exophytic soft tissue is of further aid in suggesting that this is a malignant rather than a benign process.

3

1.8 METASTASIS IN THE FEMORAL SHAFTS SECONDARY TO MULTIPLE MYELOMA

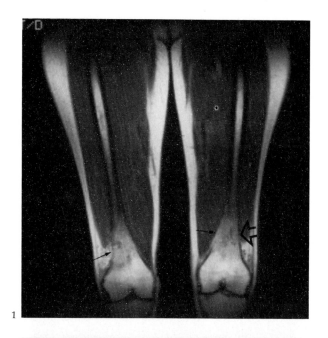

1

The patient is a 56-year-old female with known multiple myeloma. Figure 1 demonstrates replacement of the normal high-signal bone marrow, which can be seen above and below the areas of abnormality demarcated by the open arrow. The small arrows demonstrate cortical permeative, destructive changes.

Figure 2 shows a permeative and less focal pattern of infiltration, again consistent with a diffuse infiltrate of a bone marrow process (large arrow). The long-stemmed arrow also demonstrates a change in the proximal shaft below the trochanter.

The small arrows demonstrate an abnormal signal in the acetabulum on the left and suggest involvement in the proximal shaft of the right femur below the trochanters. The ability to place in the scanning gantry both sides of the body part in question facilitates the more subtle detection of possible additional areas of involvement, such as that seen in the proximal femoral shafts, versus the fairly blatant destructive change in the lower shafts.

The axial images (Figure 3) are also of help. The normal high-signal bone marrow on the right (open arrow) is easily compared to the lower signal or "dirty" appearance of the bone marrow on the left (curved arrow).

This case is through the courtesy of Dr. Robert Chiteman of Maryland Magnetic Imaging.

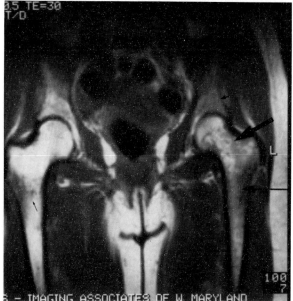

2

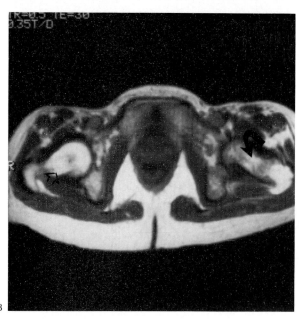

3

1.9 LIPOMA IN THE CERVICAL REGION

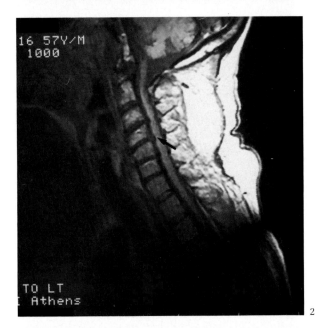

1

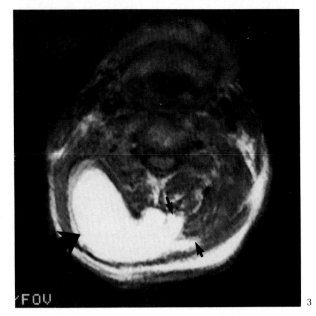

2

A 57-year-old male with a long-standing mass in the posterior side of the neck demonstrates the characteristics of a typical lipoma. On Figure 1 the upper and lower limits of the lipoma are identified (long arrows). The lipomatous content can be compared quickly to reference fat in the neck (curved arrow).

Figure 2 demonstrates spondylitic ridging and indentation in the cord at numerous levels.

Figure 3 shows the axial representation of the lipoma and its relationship to the paraspinal musculature in its fairly well-demarcated but somewhat lobulated contour. The ability to image such tumors in more than one plane, aside from demonstrating the tissue characteristic of fat, allows exclusion of a significant amount of nonfatty tissue within them. A completely homogeneous lipoma is a benign lesion. Examination of this lesion in several planes is advocated to exclude the presence of small amounts of soft tissue or fibrous strands, which may suggest a sarcomatous element. In this case the lesion was believed to be a totally benign lipoma, and its chronicity further assured its benign nature.

3

1.10 FIBROUS DYSPLASIA

Figure 1 demonstrates a large area of involvement of the intratrochanteric shaft as well as the left femoral neck. This is a T2-weighted image. The high-signal areas within the fibrous matrix probably represent a small cyst or possibly some retained fat from bone marrow that has not yet been displaced by the process.

Figure 2 demonstrates the T1 appearance. Figure 3 demonstrates the axial spin density appearance of the lesion, showing slight expansion (Figure 3b). This is typical of fibrous dysplasia, as is the low-density or fibrous appearance of the processes that replace the normal bony trabecular contents (Figure 3a). The focal sclerotic rim is identified on Figures 1 and 2 by the large arrows. This is helpful in differentiating between fibrous dysplasia and a rapidly growing neoplastic structure. Otherwise, the expansion and bulky size of the area of involvement might be considered to represent a more aggressive form of abnormality.

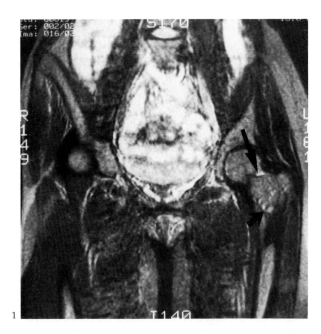

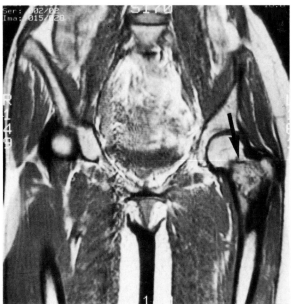

1

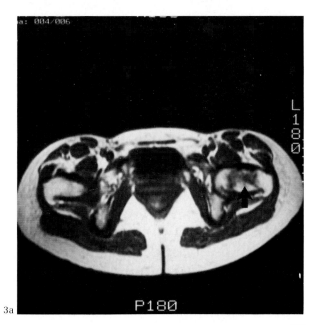

2

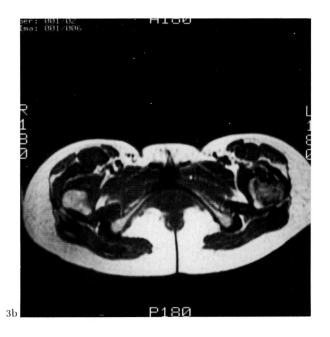

3b

3a

1.11 MULTIPLE METASTATIC LESIONS IN THE HIPS AND FEMURS

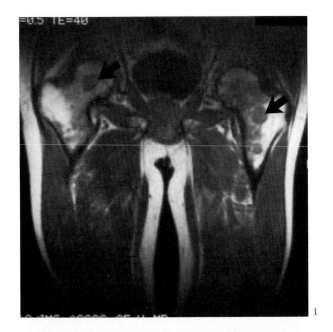

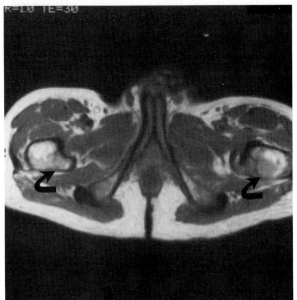

This 54-year-old female presented with fairly well-marginated, low-signal areas involving both sides of the femoral neck (Figure 1, large arrows). Figure 2, in the axial plane, confirms the decreased signal on the left in a fairly well-demarcated manner. Note the fairly normal appearance of the bone marrow on the right (curved arrow).

In Figure 3, a focal area of destruction of the cortex is nicely demonstrated by the increased signal in the normally low-signal or signal-void bony cortex. The presence of cellular material beyond the outer contour of the cortex is also suggested (Figure 3a). Figure 3b demonstrates even more focal bone destruction and exophytic extension of the metastatic material.

Figure 4 demonstrates, in a dramatic fashion, the gross destruction of the lateral aspect of the cortex of the proximal left femoral shaft. The small arrow indicates the superior level of frank cortical destruction, although immediately above the arrowhead there is also an increased signal, suggesting that some permeative destruction may be occurring. The large arrow demonstrates the outer lateral boundary of the exophytically extending material. This patient has a known adenocarcinoma, and this study was obtained to evaluate the cause of hip pain.

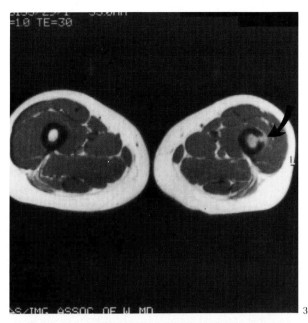

3a

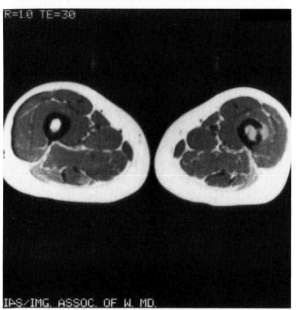

3b

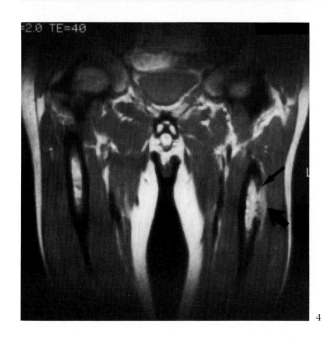

4

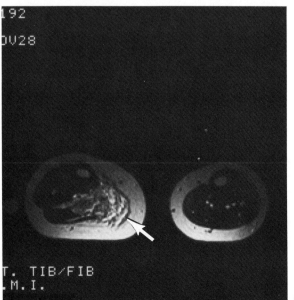

1.12 HEMANGIOMA OF THE THIGH MUSCLES

This is an 8-year-old male. Figure 1 demonstrates the replacement of the normal intermediate-signal muscle with a heterogeneous tissue mass. There are some focal, serpentine, rounded areas suggestive of large venous structures, as well as some focal areas of decreased signal consistent with calcifications. Essentially the muscle mass has been replaced rather than increased in size. Compare the axial MRI images (Figures 2a and 2b) to the computed tomography (CT) image (Figure 3). On the MRI scan, there is an abundance of information about the soft tissue structures in relation to the abnormal tissue. By contrast, the CT scan suggests some irregularity but is otherwise uninformative.

The differential diagnosis in such a case is between a hemangioma and possibly a low-grade sarcoma. The absence of increasing bulk in the abnormal muscle indicates a hemangioma or vascular process rather than a sarcoma, which is typically bulky and increases the size of the structure involved. There are various types of hemangiomas, ranging from very small, capillary hemangiomas with minimal involvement to large, aggressive mixed tumors including lymphatic arterial and venous components. However, on the basis of the MRI image alone, low-grade sarcoma cannot be excluded. It is included in the differential diagnosis of this particular case.

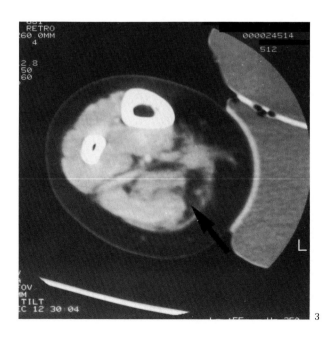

1.13 QUESTION OF RECURRENT CLEAR CELL SARCOMA IN THE THIGH

This 27-year-old female has undergone resection of a clear cell sarcoma along the medial aspect of the thigh. The distortion of the subcutaneous tissues and muscle is apparent on the coronal image (Figure 1) and the axial images (Figures 2 and 3). This soft tissue extrinsic to the muscle can be evaluated and has been followed on several different imaging sessions. There is some intermediate signal rather than the low signal expected with a simple scar, which has raised clinical concern about recurrence of the sarcoma. MRI offers an excellent way to differentiate between a scar and a recurrent tumor by providing contrast between the two types of tissues. The ability to image in more than one plane also allows more exact volumetric appreciation of the abnormal areas and of any subtle increase in volume, which may denote tumor recurrence.

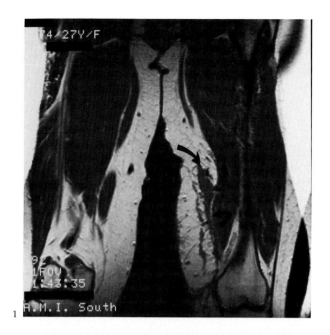

1

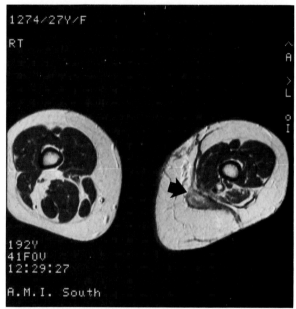

2

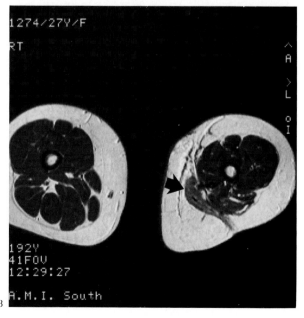

3

1.14 ILIAC METASTASIS

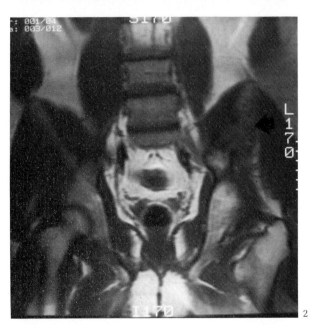

This is a 32-year-old male with a destructive lesion clearly defined on the axial CT-like image (Figure 1). The frank destruction of the iliac bone is identified (curved arrow). The extraosseous extension is also seen clearly (large arrow). Figure 2 demonstrates a coronal image and shows its relationship to the iliac bone.

Figure 3 demonstrates, in the sagittal plane, the destructive exophytic nature of this lesion.

1.15 OSTEOID OSTEOMA VERSUS SIMPLE BONE ISLAND

This is a 77-year-old male with focal, nonradicular back pain. Figures 1 and 2 are sagittal axial demonstrations of an area of focal, compact bone sclerosis. This correlates with the characteristic appearance of sclerosis and, in general appears to be a simple bone infarct or bone island (Figure 3, plain film, large arrow). However, there is a complication in that this is also the level and side of focal back pain. Some typical osteoid osteoma is represented by an osteoid focus, which appears lucent, surrounded by sclerosis of bone, reflecting the rich osteoid focus and its rich vascular supply causing enhanced bone growth at this level. Pain is secondary to the vasogenic reaction of surrounding vessels and their influence on adjacent nerves. The vascular response to aspirin also helps to provide the characteristic relief of intermittent night pain that is typical of osteoid osteoma.

Bone islands are benign, asymptomatic, dense trabecular bone growths, which can appear at any age in any bone. The differential diagnosis in such patients is, of course, osteoblastic mets.

A small nidus is not identified, and the axial and sagittal representations of this lesion help to exclude a focus, although previous case reports have stated that the osteoid focus may be radiopaque, with little or no reaction.

In general, this should be considered a bone island. The differential diagnosis is osteoid osteoma, particularly with patients who have pain in this area.

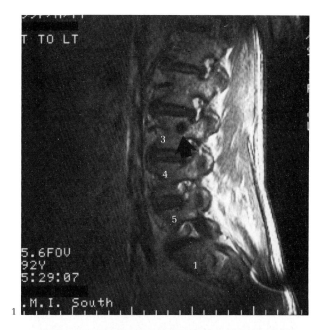

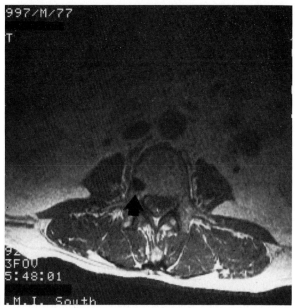

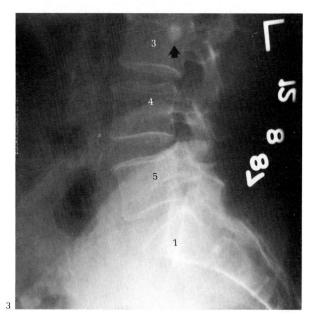

1.16 LIPOMA OF THE VASTUS MEDIALIS

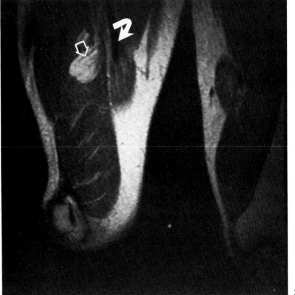

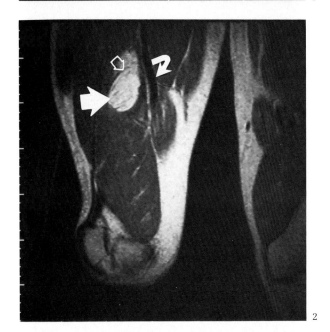

This is a 62-year-old male with a palpable, nontender mass in the thigh. A fairly well-demarcated mass with a signal intensity similar to that of subcutaneous fat is shown arising from the central portion of the vastus medialis muscle deep to the rectus femoris muscle (Figures 1 and 2, large arrows). It has an intramuscular origin, and there is muscle fiber radiating through a portion of the tumor (Figures 2 and 3, open arrows). There is always concern that tissue other than purely fatty tissue within such masses may indicate possible sarcomatous transformation. The coronal images were of assistance here, demonstrating the continuity of the muscle fibers running through the tumor in a fairly uniform fashion. This appearance suggested that these fibers represent muscle fiber rather than a sarcomatous component of the tumor mass.

On Figures 2 and 3 (curved arrows), note the visualization of the large superficial vein and the nicely demonstrated lumen, with absence of any signal suggesting patent flowing blood at this level.

1.17 LUMBAR SPINE NEUROFIBROMA

At the L2–3 level, best identified on Figures 1 and 2 by the large arrows, is a mass exiting in a dumbbell shape through the right neural foraminal canal. It shows increased signal intensity compared to the intermediate-signal roots identified by the small arrow on Figure 1. The mass is well circumscribed and can also be identified on Figure 3a in the sagittal plane. This finding and the typical dumbbell shape are consistent with a neurofibroma. These findings can be incidental but usually reflect the nerve-compressive symptoms at the level and side at which they are identified.

Note on Figure 3b the difficulty of identifying the neuroma, which shows a slightly more succulent appearance or an increase in T2-weighted characteristics and blends with the cerebrospinal fluid (CSF) at this level. We routinely obtain a spin echo with T1- and T2-weighted characteristics in the saggital plane and obtain axial T1-weighted anatomic images. On occasion, because of the different histologic makeup of various tumors, the T1- or T2-weighted images may prove helpful in increasing the conspicuity of the lesion.

Incidental note is made of the conus on Figure 3a (small arrow). This is included in most lumbar spine patients of normal size because of the improved surface coil technology and is useful for excluding unusual conus lesions that may mimic lumbar pathology.

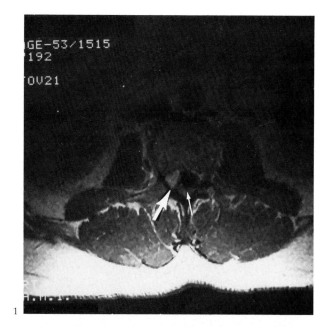

1

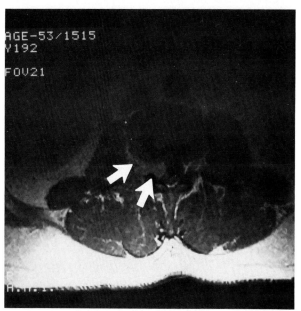

2

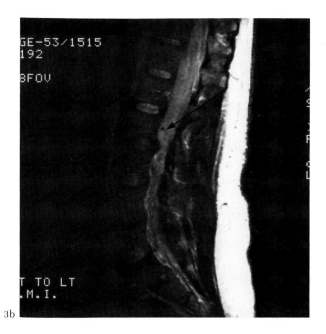

3b

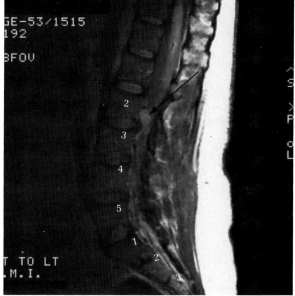

3a

1.18 METASTASIS OF THE LUMBAR SPINE IN PATIENT WITH KNOWN PROSTATE CANCER

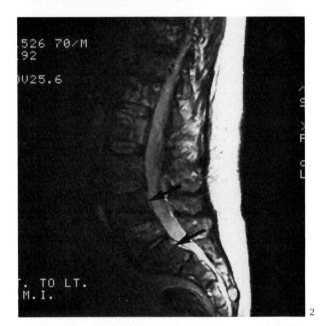

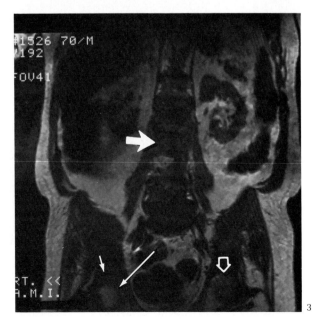

In this 70-year-old male with known prostate cancer, there is good demonstration of widespread metastatic involvement of the bones of the lumbar spine. Characteristic signal loss and altered bone marrow appearance, with almost total replacement of several vertebral bodies (Figure 1, large arrows), are noted. Collapse of the vertebral bodies with canal stenosis or cord compression can be assessed at the same time. Note in this case that almost all bone-marrow-containing cavities have been replaced with an intermediate to low signal consistent with the hypercellularity seen with metastatic disease.

Figure 2 of the T2-weighted sagittal image demonstrates nice enhancement of CSF producing a myelographic effect and allowing good assessment of the lumbar canal and exclusion of any metastatic compression or stenosis of the canal.

Figure 3, a body coil coronal scout film, also allows the opportunity to assess adjacent bony structures, such as the totally replaced bone marrow of the iliac bone on the right (small arrow) versus the normal appearance of the bone marrow cavity of the femoral head on the left (long arrow). The iliac bone marrow cavity can be compared to the more normal appearance on the left (open arrow).

1.19 LIPOMA OF THE LEFT THIGH AND QUESTION OF SARCOMA

This is a 54-year-old male with a mass in the left lateral thigh. The mass is easily identified on axial T1 and T2 images (Figures 1 and 2, large arrows). Note the excellent differentiation between the muscle tissue of the vastus lateralis in this tumor. This mass appears to be arising outside of the muscle itself. The axial images alone raise the question of whether there is damaged muscle lateral to the tumor. However, the coronal images (Figures 3a and 3b) demonstrate this to be a rounded structure with the tumor and not muscle fiber.

This tumor is predominantly fatty, and the signal change is identical to that of the subcutaneous fat of the thigh. In evaluation of lipomas, there is always concern about evaluating additional soft tissue structures within the lipoma that can suggest sarcomatous change or a sarcomatous component to the lipoma. This concern is raised with intermediate- to low-signal rounded structures, as well as with some interstitial rounded structure (designated by the white curved arrow); there is also additional interstitial stroma (Figure 3b, open arrow). Classification of lipomas can sometimes be difficult, and even tiny amounts of material other than purely fatty material should raise a suspicion of low-grade sarcomatous components.

This case is through the courtesy of Dr. M. W. Cooper and Dr. Phillip Marone at Philadelphia Magnetic Imaging.

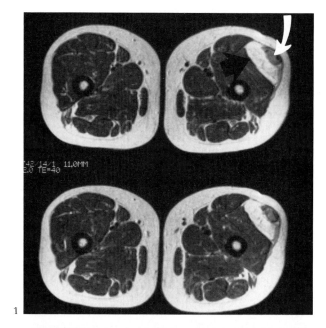

1

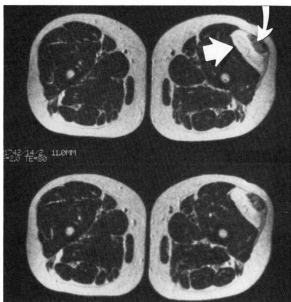

2

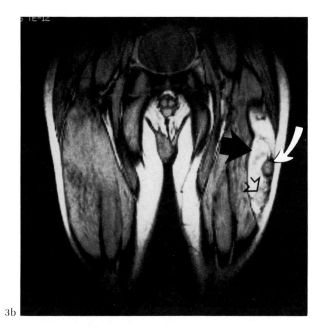

3b

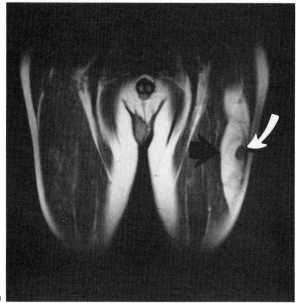

3a

1.20 FEMORAL AND PELVIC BONE METASTASES

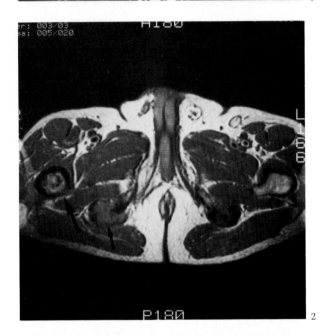

This is a 69-year-old male with a known primary cancer and right hip pain. Figure 1 demonstrates a characteristic low-density lesion associated with metastatic disease. Our experience with MRI has been that focal bone pain, even with a negative bone scan, can be best evaluated for early changes in bone marrow cellularity by MRI. The typical low density seen in replacement of normal fatty, high-signal bone marrow aids the earliest detection of metastatic disease. The metastasis is well demonstrated (large arrow). The open arrow demonstrates the slightly irregular, poorly defined medial edge of the metastasis.

Figure 2 (large arrow) demonstrates metastatic involvement and erosion of the posterior cortex of the right femoral shaft. Compare this to the left normal shaft designated by the open arrow. The small arrow demonstrates ischial metastasis on the right side.

Figure 3 demonstrates the T2-weighted characteristics of the same findings. Again, note the abnormal appearance of the bone marrow on the right (large arrow) versus the normal-appearing bone marrow on the left (open arrow). The ischial metastasis on T2 weighting shows an increase in signal.

This patient had had a previous CT scan and plain films, which were unimpressive. The patient had also undergone MRI scanning of the lumbar spine to exclude disc disease as the cause of the right hip pain. Our clinicians are now well acclimated to the use of MRI and employ it even when the bone scan is negative to exclude underlying metastatic disease as the cause of focal bone pain.

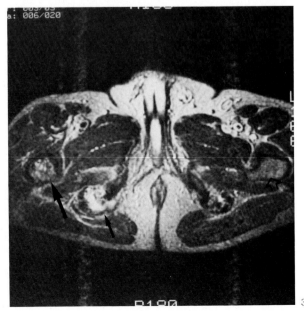

1.21 NONOSSIFYING FIBROMA

Figures 1 and 2 demonstrate the scalloped appearance of a defect in the cortex. The nonossifying fibroma is similar to a fibrous cortical defect and represents the follow-up to the defect. Fibrous defects are usually repaired in early adulthood; our patient is a 34-year-old male. This defect was discovered incidentally. The femur is at a typical location (Figure 3). There is an absence of bulging, which helps to differentiate this lesion from a chondral mixoid fibroma, and there is a more V-shaped appearance to this lesion compared to the oval shape of a chondral miscoid fibroma. There is no significant change suggesting malignancy, and the sclerotic margin is easily identified. The inner margin is usually more dense. The outer margins of these areas are thin. These lesions, like fibrous cortical defects, can regress spontaneously. They are also termed *xanthomas.*

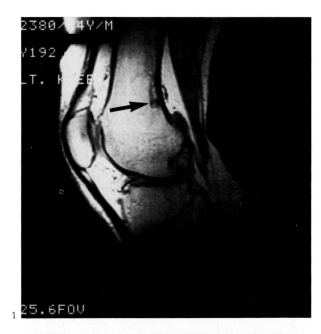

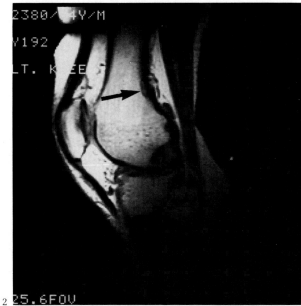

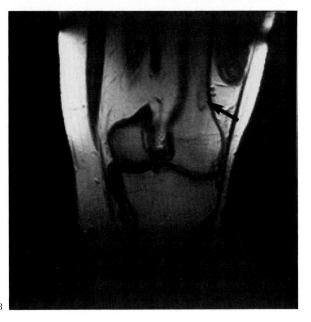

1.22 ENCHONDROMA

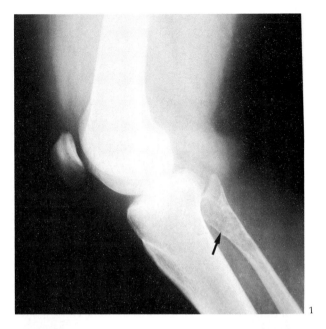

1

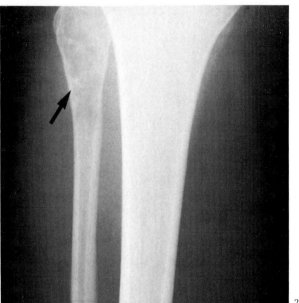

2

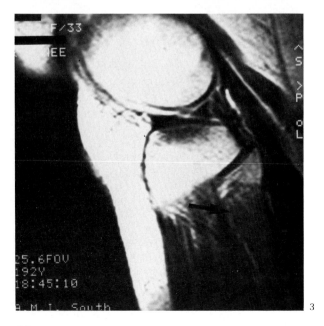

3

This is a 33-year-old female with an incidental abnormality in the knee. The characteristic intramedullary lesion in the proximal fibular shaft is identified on Figures 1 and 2 by large arrows. There is a ground glass appearance with at least some stippled calcification. There is intramedullary expansion along the long axis of the abnormality. This is consistent with an enchondroma. Figure 3 correlates nicely with the lateral film, again demonstrating the intramedullary process in the noncontinuity of the lesion with the outer cortex. Figure 4 correlates nicely with the plain film (Figure 2). The matrix on the T1-weighted Figures (4a and 4b) is low signal and is difficult to differentiate from fibrous dysplasia; in fact, giant cell, unicameral bone cyst, and fibrous dysplasia are the differential diagnoses for this lesion. Enchondromas are usually seen in the hand and wrist, but every bone except the skull can be involved. Location in the long bones tends to make this more prone to malignancy, and pain is usually the sign of malignant transformation. The enchondroma grows from within the medullary canal.

Treatment includes curettage and bone graft. The MR scan demonstrates nicely the entire extent of involvement of the bone in the fibula head on Figures 1 and 4, and the full extent necessary for curettage of the entire lesion can be well identified with MRI.

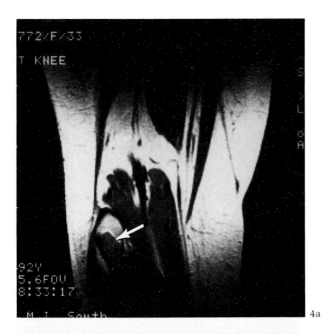

4a

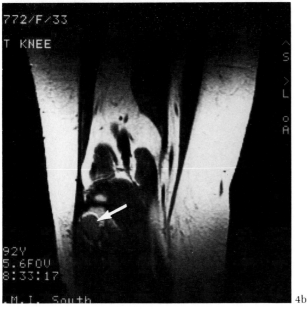

4b

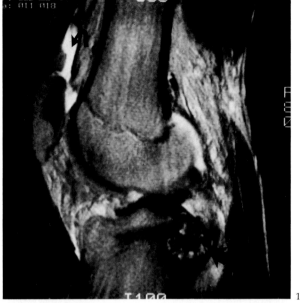

1.23 CHONDROBLASTOMA

This is a well-demarcated 1.5- to 2-cm mass that is roughly rounded and composed of a mixed matrix of both increased signal, representing cartilage, and decreased signal, representing calcification. It is located in the epiphyseal line, which is a tremendous aid to the diagnosis of the chondroblastoma. The patient is a 16-year-old male, and these tumors are commonly seen before the cessation of chondral bone growth. They are also most often seen in males. Figure 1 is a sagittal cut through the lesion demarcated by the large arrow. There is also a small joint effusion (curved arrow) that correlates nicely with the plain film (Figure 2). Figure 3 is a representation of the tumor. The large arrow points to the well-demarcated, sclerotic edge, and the long arrow points to calcifications within the matrix typical of the chondroblastoma.

A CT scan demonstrates the lesion in the proximal tibia (Figure 4). There is also evidence of a small amount of calcification (small arrow), although more detail of the matrix is available by MRI.

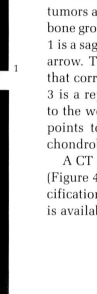

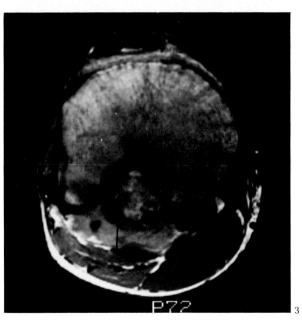

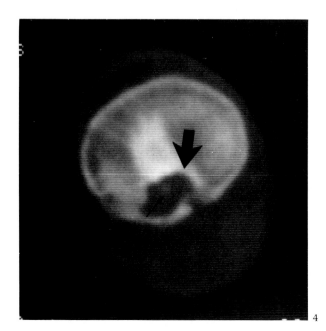

1.24 NONOSSIFYING FIBROMA

This knee in a young adult was evaluated for internal derangement, and a lesion along the cortical shaft of the distal femoral shaft was noted. This represents a benign lesion of bone called a *nonossifying* or *nonosteogenic fibroma*. The smaller lesions with a similar appearance are also known as *benign cortical defects*. The thin but complete cortical margin and the cortical location are nicely demonstrated. There is a slight cortical bulging best seen on the sagittal images (Figures 1 and 2, large arrow). The complete sclerotic rim is also well identified (Figure 3, curved arrow).

These defects are considered to represent a fault in ossification. They can enlarge and are susceptible to fracture, but are otherwise considered benign. The location in long bones is considered typical.

The most common location, as demonstrated by this case, is the lower shaft of the femur. The lesions can be found in the end of any of the long bones and have also been reported in the flat bones.

Because of the bulging and the slight enlargement of such a lesion, the diagnosis of chondromyscoid fibroma should also be considered.

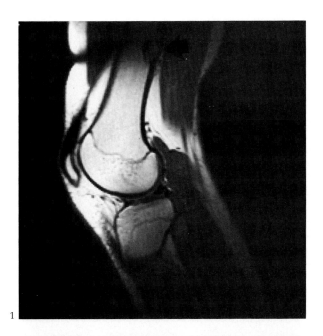

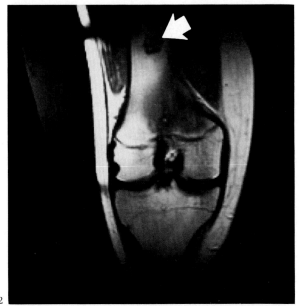

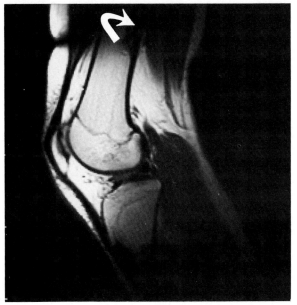

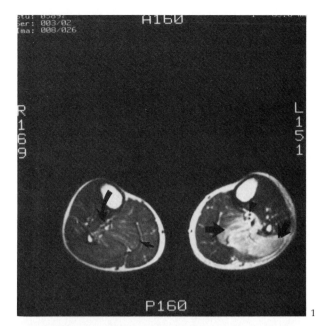

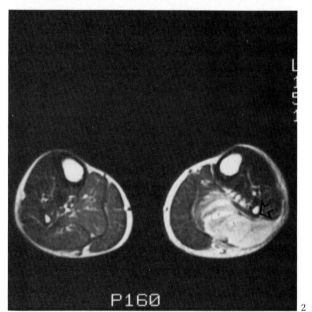

1.25 KAPOSI SARCOMA

This is a 45-year-old male with known acquired immuno-deficiency syndrome (AIDS) and a nontender, enlarging mass in the left calf. The distinct alteration of the signal identifies the abnormal muscle. The evidence of enlarging muscle mass, particularly in light of the clinical finding of a nontender, enlarging mass, all aid in the easy diagnosis of a muscle tumor, in this case a Kaposi sarcoma. There is excellent evidence of the muscles that are involved and good definition of the spared muscles, as well as sparing of the bony cortex. The abnormal muscle is outlined by arrows and is slightly enlarged compared to the normal left side. Without the clinical knowledge that this mass is not tender, it would be difficult to exclude a simple myositis on the basis of the available images.

On Figure 1, note the involvement of the lateral head of the gastrocnemius as well as the soleus muscle. On the unaffected right side, a small arrow demonstrates the tendon of the semimembranous muscle that nicely separates the medial and lateral heads of the gastrocnemius muscle. Also note the ease of identifying the popliteal artery, vein and the tibial nerve on both the unaffected side (curved arrow) and the affected side to even better effect (arrowhead).

On Figure 2 (open arrowhead), also note the excellent visualization of the cortex by a negative or a signal void and the good definition of the noninvolvement of bony structures with this abnormality.

On Figure 3, several dilated veins are identified. The reversed flow of the veins and their somewhat slow flow allow enhancement (arrowhead).

Figure 4 demonstrates a relative lack of asymmetry, as well as a slight, nonspecific swelling and a slight increase in signal on the T1-weighted images (arrowheads outline the abnormal muscle mass).

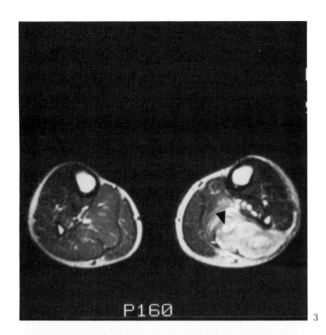

P160

3

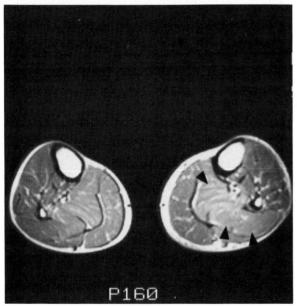

P160

4

33

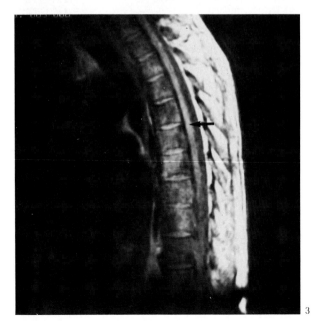

1.26 METASTATIC BONE TUMOR SECONDARY TO PRIMARY TESTICULAR CANCER

This is a 33-year-old male with a primary testicular cancer. There is extensive metastatic disease, but of importance for orthopedics is the demonstration of bony metastasis. The usual underlying process of increased cellularity that displaces the bone marrow and fat causes a decrease in signal, which is believed to be typical and representative of metastatic disease (small arrows, Figure 1). The sparing of a portion of the fat and bone marrow is also identified at the L4 level (large arrow). Note that the assessment of compression of the vertebral bodies is easily made.

On Figure 2, the extensive amount of metastatic disease, particularly into the lower sacral and coccygeal segments, often not included in routine CT scans of the lumbar spine, is demonstrated (small arrowhead).

Incidental metastatic disease to the bladder is also nicely shown on the sagittal views through the pelvis (curved arrow, Figure 1).

In addition, sagittal images can be used to survey the entire cord and to exclude any cord compression at any level from C1 through the sacral region. Note the ease of visualization of the cord in this noninvasive technique (small arrow, Figure 3).

1.27 LIPOMA OF THE RIGHT THIGH

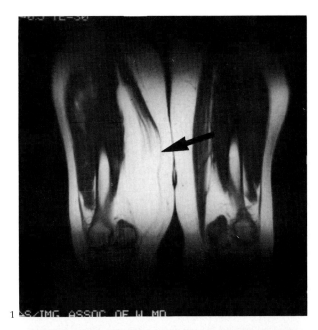

Sagittal, axial, and coronal views demonstrate a well-circumscribed, high-signal-intensity mass arising immediately medial to and possibly involving a portion of the vastus medialis muscle. This mass displaces and may also be partially involving and arising from the gracilis muscle. Note the small capsule separating this predominantly fatty tumor from the subcutaneous tissues of the thigh. Findings are most consistent with a benign lipoma.

In addition to typifying the contents of a tumor such as this lipoma, the ability to image this mass in the sagittal and coronal planes gives a more true appreciation of the overall total size and volume of such tumors (Figures 1 and 3). The involvement, or rather apparent lack of involvement of the surrounding bone and musculature (Figure 2), is also helpful in separating benign from malignant soft tissue neoplasms. This is the characteristic appearance of a lipoma. The only differential diagnosis with a mass of this high signal intensity is an acute hematoma.

This case is through the courtesy of Dr. Robert Chiteman of Maryland Magnetic Imaging.

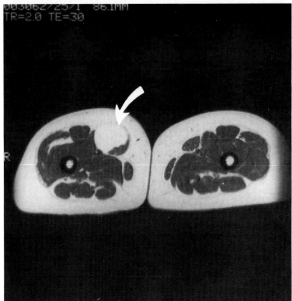

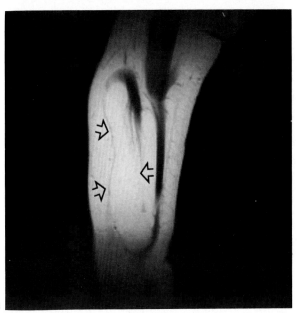

1.28 FIBROUS DYSPLASIA

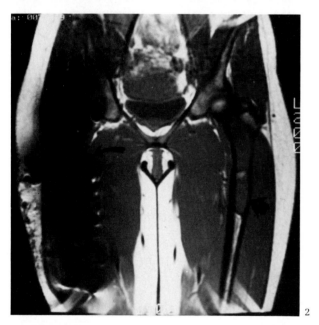

1

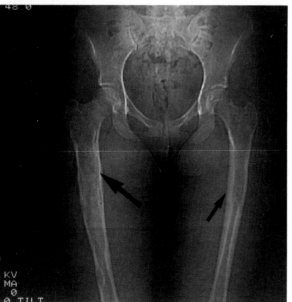

2

3

In this 18-year-old female, the right bone shaft was previously repaired for fibrous dysplasia; the left bone shaft was evaluated and also shows the characteristic findings associated with fibrous dysplasia. This dysplasia reflects fibrous replacement of a portion of the medullary cavity of bone secondary to mesenchymal abnormality. Approximately 40 percent of these patients will undergo fracture in lesions through the long bones. The radiologic features, which are also identified on the MRI scan, include expansion of the medullary canal within cortex. There is usually a lucent or thinned cortex. A later fracture through this area of the bone may respond with thickening. The characteristic location in the long bones is exhibited nicely on Figures 1 and 2 (large arrows).

Incidental note is made of the metal artifact from the placement of a plate and screws for fixation of a fracture through the right femoral shaft.

Figure 3 demonstrates the plain film findings involving both femoral shafts in a fairly characteristic fashion. The MRI scan was obtained to ascertain the extent of involvement of the left femoral shaft and demonstrates this quite well.

On Figure 4a there is evidence of the inner face between the normal bone marrow and that of the fibrous tissue-filled cavity (the long arrow with the shaft designates the normal marrow, and the small arrow within the medullary cavity demonstrates the inner face between the fibrous tissue and the bone marrow). The open-ended arrows demonstrate, in the axial plain, the extension of the shaft, as well as thinning of the cortex (Figure 4b). Figure 5 illustrates the ability of MRI to also demonstrate the inner face of the bone marrow with the characteristic fibrous cavity. The open arrow designates the fibrous cavity and slightly thin cortex on the left, and the closed small arrow demonstrates normal bone marrow with its high signal interfacing the fibrous cavity.

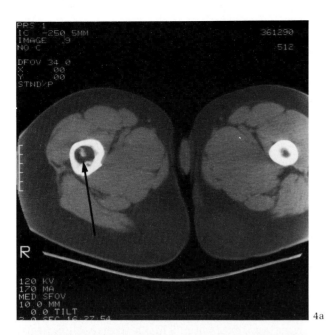

4a

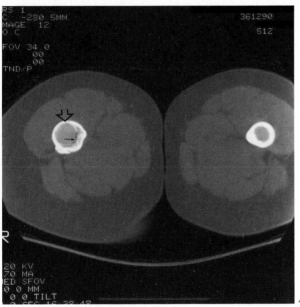

4b

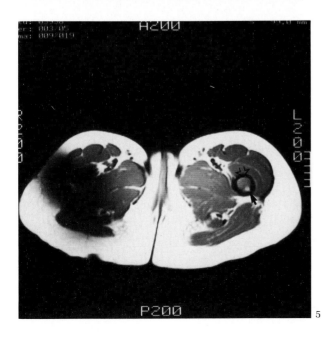

5

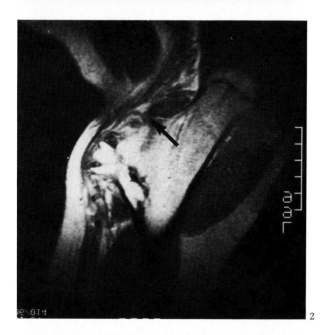

1

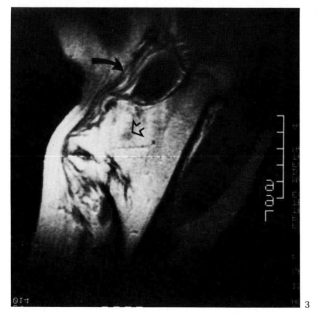

3

1.29 OSTEOCHONDROMA IN THE LEFT HUMERUS

This is a 12-year-old female with a mass in the left humerus. This mass demonstrates focal enlargement of the cortex with well-defined margins and confluence of the cortex with the normal cortex above from the proximal humeral shaft. For purposes of orientation, the large arrow on Figure 1 points to the epithesial plate of the humerus, and the small arrow points to the deltoid. The large arrows on Figures 1 and 2 demonstrate the contiguous nature of the cortex from the normal shaft into this area of enlargement. The open arrow on Figure 3 demonstrates the similar matrix of the tumorous extension. This is an osteochondroma secondary to a hypoplastic bone disturbance and believed to originate from ectopic cartilage of the growth plate. A differential demonstration can usually be made of a cartilaginous cap over the osteochondroma. These caps are believed to be congenital lesions; however, pain and rapid growth raise the suspicion of malignant transformation.

Incidentally, note that the nerves from the brachial plexus are slightly displaced as they leave the axilla and enter the upper forearm (see Figure 3, curved arrow).

Figure 4 is a plain film demonstrating the correlation between the plain film of the upper extremity and the MRI scan.

Figure 5 demonstrates that the cartilaginous cap is nicely accentuated on the T2-weighted images (curved arrow points to the cartilaginous cap of the osteochondroma).

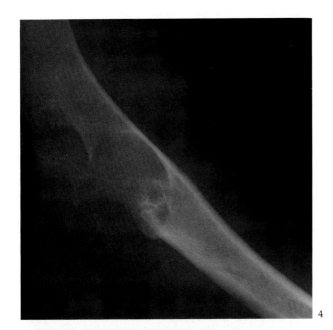

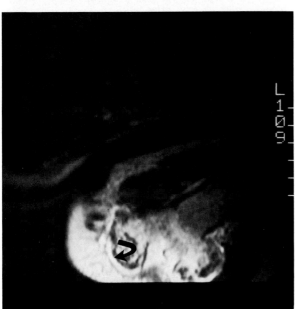

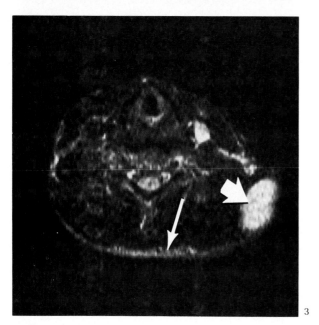

1.30 LIPOMA ARISING FROM THE LEFT TRAPEZIUS MUSCLE

This is a patient with a palpable mass in the left side (Figure 1). The coronal and axial views all demonstrate a well-defined, high-signal structure that maintains slight increase in signal on both T1 and T2 weighting (the arrows in Figures 2 and 3 designates the lipoma). The signal is roughly the same as that of the subcutaneous fat (see the arrow with the long shaft pointing to normal subcutaneous fat in the posterior neck). The lack of any internal signal alteration and the well-defined margins identify this as a lipoma. Its maintenance of signal intensity similar to that of the subcutaneous fat also helps to exclude the possibility of hematoma. These lesions are usually benign and incidental. They should, however, be scrutinized for any evidence of alteration of the homogeneous lipomatous matrix for any suggestion of a low-grade liposarcoma, which can be difficult to exclude.

1.31 OSTEOCHONDROMA OF THE FIBULA

This is an incidental mass detected on examination for trauma to the knee. It is consistent with expansion and a hypoplastic response to the cortex of the fibular shaft and represents an osteochondroma (Figures 1 and 2, arrow). Figure 3 demonstrates (open arrow), the cartilaginous cap. Although these lesions represent a congenital rest of cartilage, at times these can become painful. Pain can be a symptom of malignant transformation. This is a typical location for these lesions, and they are often detected as incidental findings on emergency room films reviewing lower extremities for fracture.

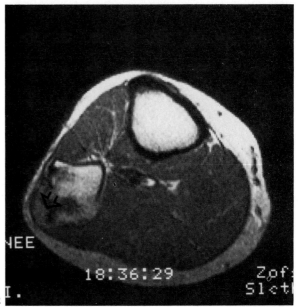

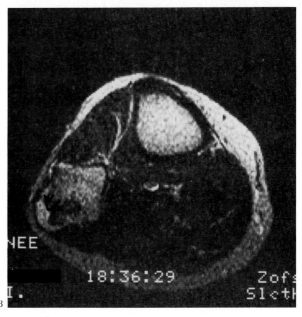

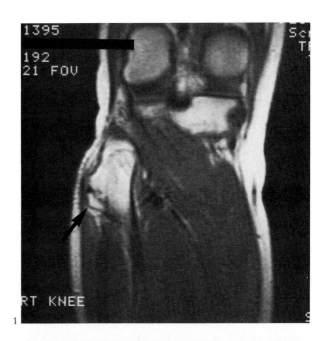

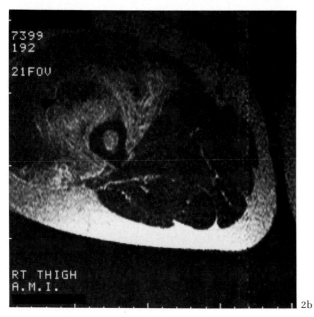

1.32 TRAUMA WITH TORN VASTUS INTERMEDIUS MUSCLE

This patient with a history of trauma presents with a painful thigh, and the disruption of the entire vastus intermedius muscle is nicely displayed on T1-weighted images (Figures 1, 3a, and 3b). The T2-weighted images on Figures 2a and 2b demonstrate partial muscle bundles floating within the edematous matrix of blood and edema in the middle thigh compartment (see arrowheads; long arrows on Figures 1a and 2 demonstrate the hematoma within the lateral bundles of a portion of the vastus muscle). Without a history of trauma, the differentiation between a primary muscle tumor and traumatic rupture of the muscle in some cases can be difficult. However, the demonstration of disruption of the normal anatomy rather than an infiltrative process (i.e., the demonstration of floating intact muscle bundles) is helpful in making this diagnosis.

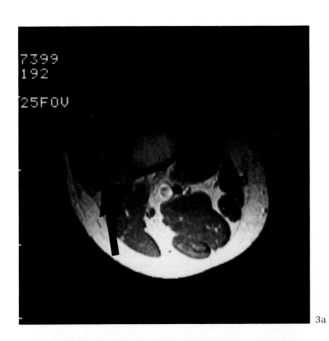

3a

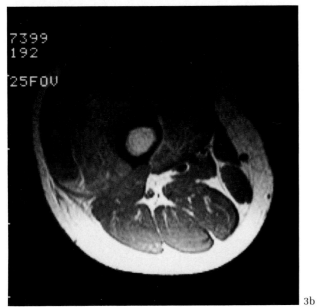

3b

43

1.33 EXOSTOSIS OF THE PROXIMAL FIBULA

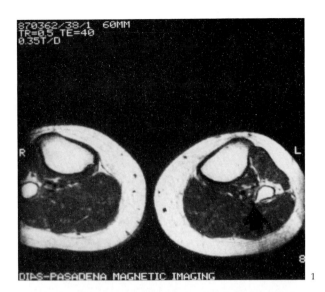

1

This is a 42-year-old female with a small exostosis discovered incidentally. Figure 1 is a comparison of axial images through the proximal fibula demonstrating a small bony outgrowth consistent with a tiny osteochondroma. Proton and slightly T2-weighted images also confirm the regular nature of the cortex, suggesting a tiny cartilaginous cap and absence of any malignant features (arrowheads point to the exostosis on Figures 2 and 3).

This case is through the courtesy of Dr. M. Shah and Dr. Rodolfo A. Lopez of Pasadena Magnetic Imaging.

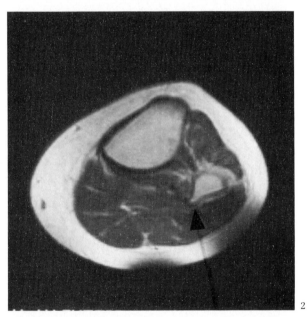

2

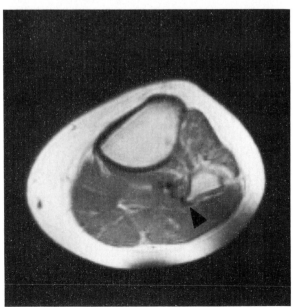

3

1.34 OSTEOCHONDROMA OF THE TIBIA

This is a 13-year-old female with a palpable mass. Figures 1a and 1b demonstrate a solitary exostosis or osteochondroma projecting from the posterior aspect of the distal tibia. The cartilaginous cap is believed to be present on Figures 2 and 3 (large arrows). The continuity of the lesion with the cortex is well identified on these images (see curved arrows of Figures 1 and 2). These benign bone lesions can develop bursae and can become painful secondary to irritation. Pain and continued growth after puberty can also be a sign of malignant degeneration. These lesions, when malignant, usually degenerate into chondrosarcomas. MRI evaluation should be able to demonstrate the loss of the normal benign features of an osteochondroma.

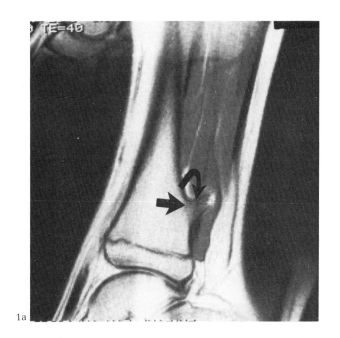

1a

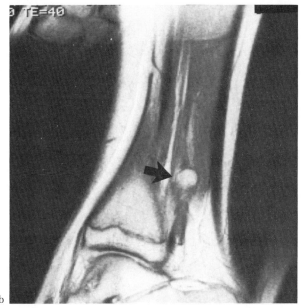

1b

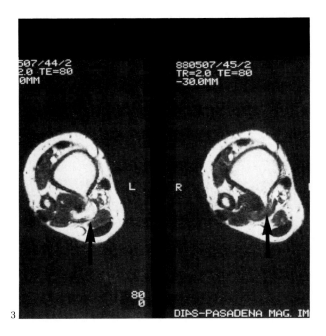

3

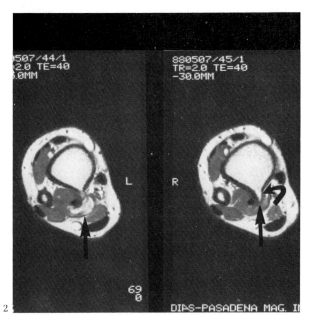

2

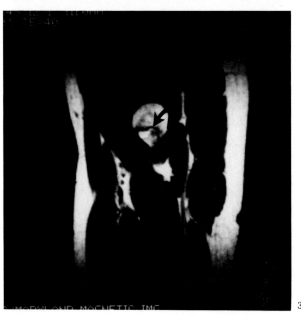

1.35 BONE CYST, SOLITARY VERSUS HEMORRHAGIC CYST

This is a 36-year-old male with pain in the hip who has a cystic lesion with a fairly well-deformed, sclerotic margin. This lesion does not expand into the soft tissues, and the matrix shows increased signal on all imaging parameters, including T1 proton density and T2, suggesting high-protein, possibly old hemorrhagic content. There is also evidence on Figure 1 (small arrowhead), of a small fragment in the dependent portion of the cyst, suggesting a fallen fragment from previous trauma to the now thinned cortex of the cyst. The cyst appears to be parallel with the long axis of the neck.

This appears to represent a cystic deformity within bone; the differential diagnosis is between a simple bone cyst and a hemorrhagic cyst. This lesion does not have the expanded or blown-out appearance of an aneurysmal bone cyst, although the location is good for a possible aneurysmal cyst; this possibility cannot be totally excluded.

Solitary bone cysts usually are believed to be secondary to overreactive osteoclasts with obstruction to interstitial fluid drainage; 75 percent of these lesions occur in the humerus or femur. The features previously described are also typical of a solitary bone cyst.

Small amounts of hemorrhage into a cyst can occur, particularly with prior minimal trauma. Hemorrhagic cysts cannot be totally excluded and are also of concern because of the high signal within the cyst content. We can safely exclude fibrous dysplasia. The fibrous matrix demonstrated in other cases in this collection is unlike the matrix demonstrated here, which has an increased signal on all parameters.

The large arrows on Figures 1 and 2 demonstrate the thin, sclerotic margin and the nonexpansile characteristic of this oval-shaped mass. The arrowhead demonstrates what appears to be a small bone fragment in the dependent portion of the cyst on Figure 1. On Figure 3, the curved arrow again demonstrates the well-defined, sclerotic margin and high signal seen in the sagittal plane through this cystic abnormality. Note also that the sagittal and coronal views allow demonstration of the nonexpansile character of this cystic abnormality.

This case is through the courtesy of Dr. Robert Chiteman of Maryland Magnetic Imaging.

1.36 OSTEOCHONDROMAS

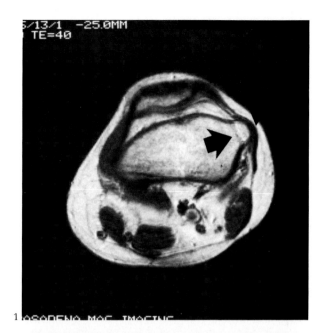

This is a 10-year-old female with a mass arising from the lateral aspect of the femur. Figures 1 and 2, representing T1- and T2-weighted images in the axial plane through the lesion, demonstrate a structure that shows good confluence of the normal cortex with the well-defined mass, which has an overall benign appearance and is typical of an osteochondroma. Curved arrows in Figures 1 and 2 demonstrate displacement of the lateral retinaculum and muscle tendon secondary to the osteochondroma. This abnormal protuberance makes the overlying soft tissue susceptible to injury, and a bursal sac can develop over the osteochondroma and provide a source of pain from chronic irritation as well. Figure 3 (large arrow), demonstrates a separation of the normal spongiosum from the tumerous matrix, which shows a slight increase in signal intensity. Figure 4, a T1-weighted image in the coronal plane, also demonstrates nicely the anatomic appearance of this lesion.

This case is through the courtesy of Dr. M. Dan Boone and Dr. Rodolfo A. Lopez of Pasadena Magnetic Imaging.

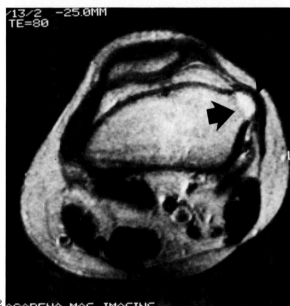

1

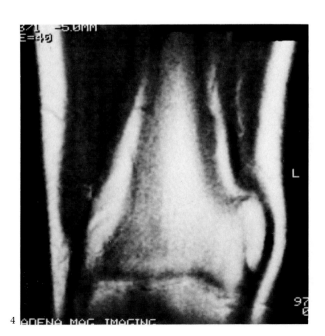

2

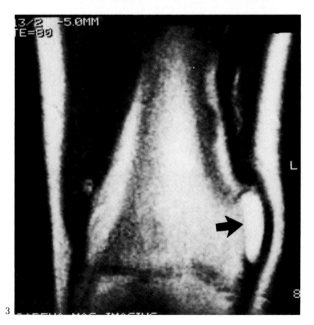

3

4

1.37 RIGHT SACRAL METASTASIS VERSUS CHONDROSARCOMA

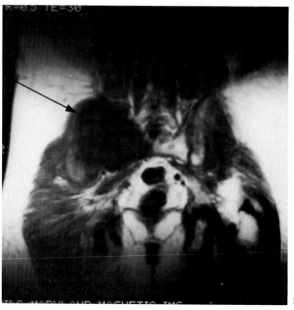

This is a 65-year-old male. Figure 1 demonstrates a tumor that appears to arise from the region of the sacroiliac joint (curved arrow). The tumor extends beyond the osseous confines of the sacral and iliac bones, which are both involved. There is also tumor eruption into the subcutaneous tissues (Figure 2, open arrow). Unlike a normal metastasis, this demonstrates a large amount of extraosseous growth, and the tumor shows a high signal on the T2-weighted images (Figure 3a; see also the T1-weighted images on Figures 3a and 3b). The excellent anatomic delineation of the tumor in each of the three orthogonal planes assists in determining the more specific appearance of the tumor. This is not clinically associated with any evidence of infection and the fat muscle plane is well preserved, even in close proximity to the tumor itself (see Figure 2, curved arrow). Increased signal on the T2-weighted images suggests that underlying cartilaginous stroma may exist. Most chondrosarcomas are found in the pelvis, involving the sacrum or pubic rami, femur, humerus, or tibia. They may not have an associated sclerotic edge. Most of the features in this case also fit a metastatic lesion, with the exception of the fairly homogeneous increase in signal on the T2-weighted images.

1

2

3a

3b

1.38 ENCHONDROMA OF THE HUMERUS

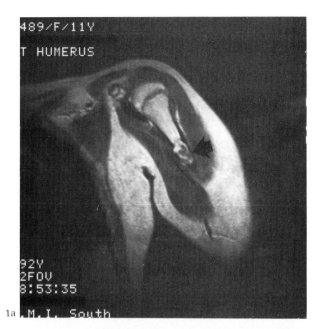

This is an 11-year-old female with a slightly expansile lesion identified on Figures 1a and 1b. The cortex is thinned and expanded in the anterior direction (see Figure 2, large arrow). The T2-weighted images (Figure 1b) demonstrate a cartilaginous matrix with bone within the defect. These features are consistent with enchondroma. This correlates well with the plain film (Figure 3).

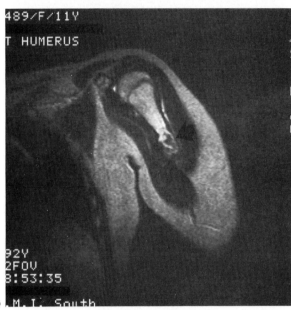

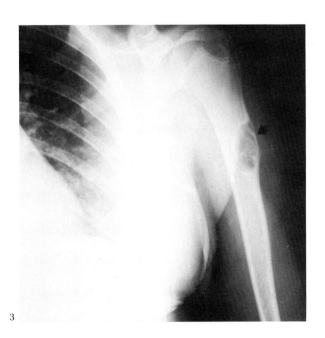

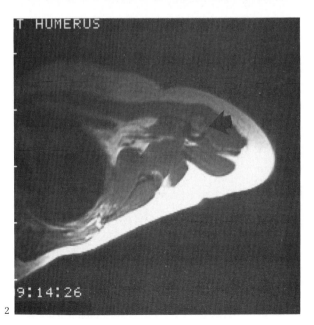

1.39 LARGE NEUROFIBROMA OF THE TIBIAL NERVE

This 46-year-old male with a nontender mass was studied with MRI. The scan demonstrates a well-circumscribed, homogeneous structure that has signal characteristics similar to those of neurofibromas seen in the spine and cranial regions (Figures 1 and 2). This is extrinsic to the bone and muscle, and the well-shaped edges and extrinsic appearance suggest that it arises from outside the muscle. This allows exclusion of a primary muscle tumor such as a rhabdomyosarcoma. Well-formed edges also help in the diagnosis of a more benign lesion. The axial images also demonstrate nicely the numerous septal compartments of the calf and are well demonstrated by MRI. Figure 3 is a T1-weighted image. Figure 4 is a T2-weighted image through the neurofibroma.

This case is through the courtesy of Dr. Robert Chiteman of Maryland Magnetic Imaging.

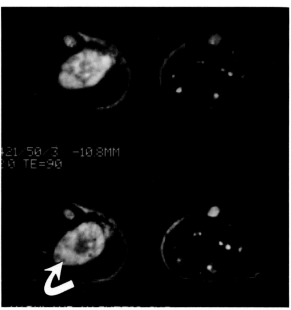

50

1.40 GIANT CELL TUMOR OF THE TIBIA

This 52-year-old male has a large, destructive lesion in the proximal end of the tibia. The cortex is broken, as demonstrated on Figures 1 and 2 by the open arrows. Figure 3 is a sagittal cut through the tumor (large arrow). The tumor is a mononuclear stromal cell that fuses to form a giant cell. It is a predominantly destructive lesion and can break the cortex, as demonstrated in this case. These lesions are generally seen in older adults, and most are identified in the metaphysis near the fused epiphyseal line.

These tumors can be classified as grade I, II, or III. Grade III represents clearly malignant tumor, most bone tumors fall into grades I or II. The appearance of this tumor, particularly with the cortical disruption, suggests malignant behavior.

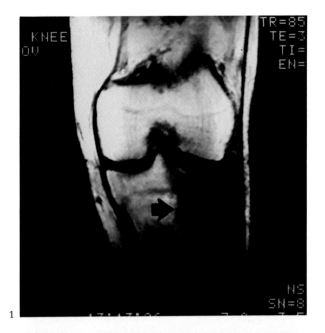

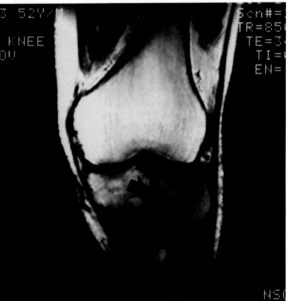

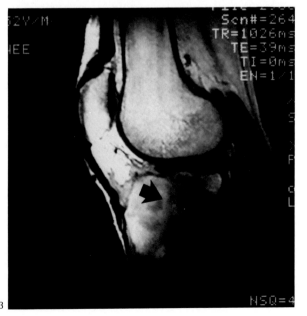

1.41 SARCOMA OF THE DISTAL CALF

This 13-year-old female demonstrates a palpable, nontender soft tissue mass posterior to the ankle that has signal characteristics similar to those of the muscle of the posterior calf. However, this mass, although very organized and discrete, extends down into a space normally occupied only by fat and the Achilles tendon (Figures 1a and 1b).

The sagittal image on Figure 2 and the large arrow demonstrate the extension of what appears to be a predominantly muscle-type mass. The absence of any extension into the associated tendon, bone, and subcutaneous tissues indicates a slightly more benign classification of sarcoma, although this is not a practically useful classification.

Figure 3 (open arrows) is a coronal image through the tumor. Note the very subtle asymmetry in this plane.

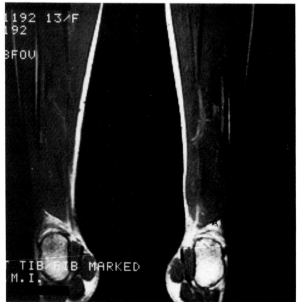

1.42 SYNOVIAL TUMOR OF THE KNEE

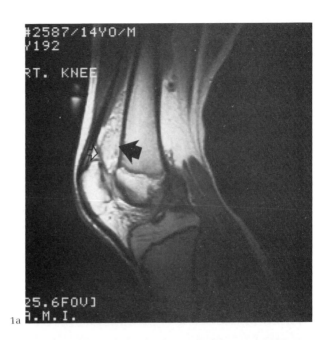

1a

An intra-articular mass is nicely identified on the sagittal views (large arrow, Figures 1a and 1b), and the intra-articular location is clearly demonstrated on the axial images. There is good demonstration of the borders of the tumor (open arrows, Figures 1 to 3). The differential diagnosis is primarily a synovial tumor, possibly a primary synovioma versus a synovial sarcoma. Pigmented villonodular synovitis should also be included. In addition, this location and the characteristic high signal intensity with an interstitial structure suggestive of capillary and possibly some lymphatic structure could be consistent with a hemangioma (long arrow, Figure 1b). The entirely intra-articular location demonstrated on the sagittal and axial images is of assistance in demonstrating the contact of the tumor with the synovium. The remainder of the structures of the knee were examined, and no additional masses were seen.

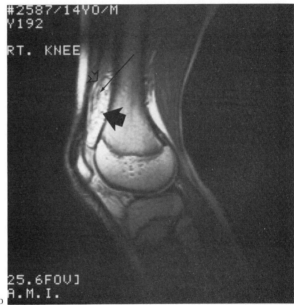

1b

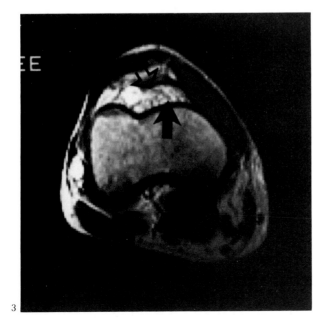

3

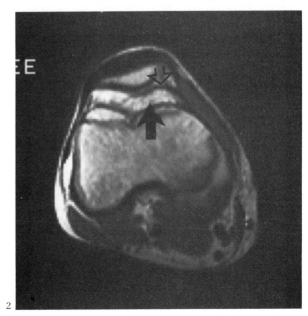

2

1.43 CALF HEMANGIOMA

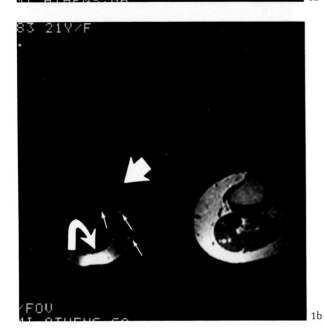

1a

1b

This 21-year-old female with a painful enlargement of the calf on MRI demonstrates asymmetric enlargement of the soft tissues in the medial subcutaneous tissues on the right (Figures 1a and 1b, large arrows). Also within this predominantly fatty stroma are numerous linear markings representing vascular element (Figures 2a and 2b, long arrows, and Figure 1b, tiny arrows). This represents a hemangioma with a predominantly fatty stroma.

Figure 1b (curved arrow) demonstrates shading artifact from the proximity of the surface coil to the posterior soft tissues of the right thigh and is not consistent with true underlying abnormality.

Figure 3 demonstrates a sagittal cut through the hemangioma. Small arrows identify vascular structures within the stroma.

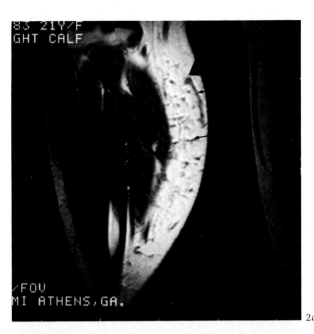

2a

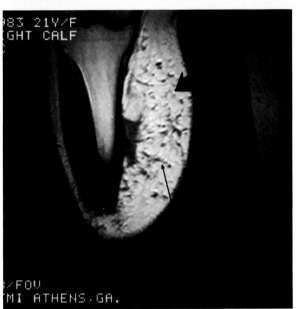

2b

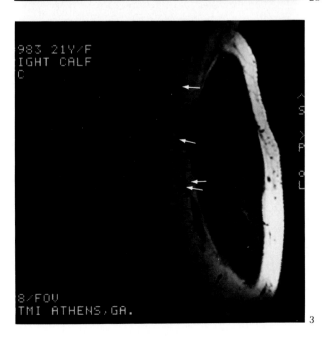

3

1.44 OSTEOPETROSIS

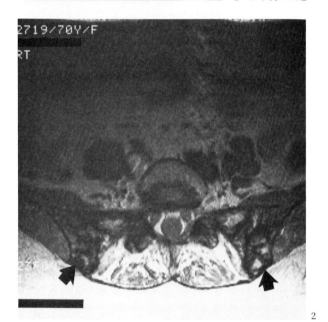

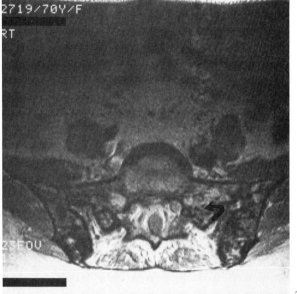

This 70-year-old female was evaluated for pain in the back associated with breast cancer. However, the patient related a history of having unusually dense bones and of being told about this since young adulthood.

The characteristic symmetric, sclerotic appearance of the bones at each level is consistent with osteopetrosis. Note the sagittal images demonstrating the unusual sclerosis around the basilar vertebral channel (Figure 1, large arrows).

The more characteristic appearance of the sacral and iliac bone is identified on Figures 2 and 3. The osteopetrosis shown on these films demonstrates an increase in the trabecular markings diffusely. In such patients, it would be extremely difficult to exclude underlying malignant change, and osteopetrosis has sometimes been linked to a premalignant state. The appearance on MRI is nonspecific, and without the patient's history of prior long-standing knowledge of this disease, it would be difficult to exclude metastatic disease.

Figure 3 (curved arrow) demonstrates the thickened trabecula in the sacrum. Figure 2 demonstrates the thickening of the trabecular markings and cortex in the iliac bone.

1.45 RIGHT TIBIAL METASTASIS

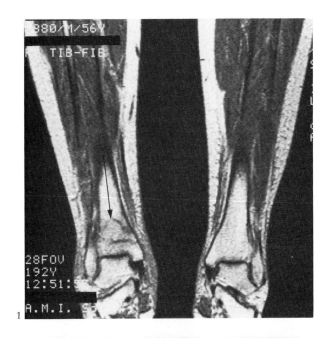

This 56-year-old male with a known primary cancer complained of right focal ankle pain and did not have a significant history of trauma. This MRI scan demonstrates a characteristic low-density lesion that is fairly well demarcated (Figure 1, long-stemmed arrow). The altered signal in a patient with known cancer makes the diagnosis of metastatic disease fairly certain. The margins in this area of involvement are poorly defined (Figures 2a and 2b, long-stemmed and large arrows).

Axial cuts through this area again confirm the malignant nature, with demonstration of cortical erosion (Figure 3, large white arrow) versus the normal intact cortex of the left extremity at the same level (open arrow).

Another differential diagnosis in this location is giant cell tumor, particularly with a closed epiphyseal plate. However, with the history of known cancer, metastatic disease is the primary choice.

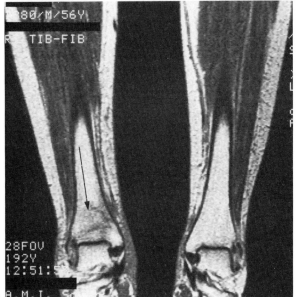

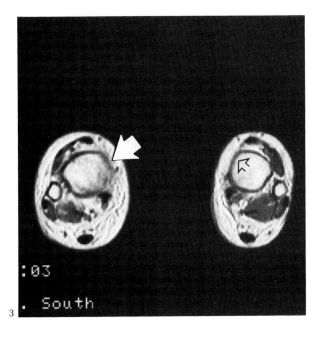

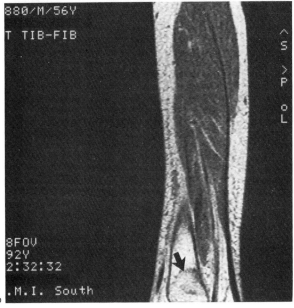

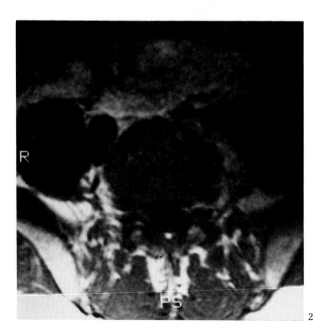

1a

1b

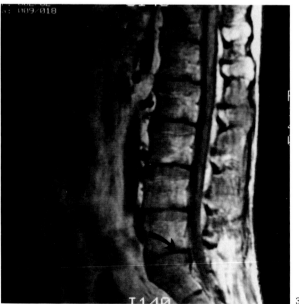

2

3

1.46 PARADISCAL MASS CONSISTENT WITH METASTASIS

This 48-year-old male had left-sided symptoms, and a CT scan (Figure 1a) demonstrated a slight bulge of the annulus. An MRI scan demonstrated a definite paradiscal mass with a signal characteristic different from that of the annulus and disc material (Figure 1b and Figure 2, large arrow). This mass was biopsied. The patient also had evidence of other bone metastatic lesions, but bony metastasis was revealed by bone scan.

This demonstrates fairly dramatically the sensitivity of MRI compared to CT. Even with a high-grade CT scan, the mass appears to represent nothing more than a disc bulge. On the MRI scan, clear contrast tissue differences allow evaluation of a definite mass.

Figure 3 demonstrates a sagittal T1-weighted image. There was no evidence on this or multiple other images to indicate any significant disc abnormality or bulge.

1.47 METASTATIC DISEASE RIGHT ILIAC BONE

In this 65-year-old female, a focal area of signal decrease in the marrow of the right iliac bone shows the significant features of a metastatic lesion. The replacement of the normal high signal of fat and bone marrow in this area demonstrates nicely the metastatic involvement (Figures 1a and 1b). On the left, concern was raised about a possible lesion superior to the acetabulum (Figure 1a, long arrow). However, on Figure 2, axial cuts through this region demonstrate this to be volume averaging of the iliac bone with the iliopsoas muscle, and there is no asymmetry to suggest underlying metastatic disease (open arrows demonstrate normal bone bilaterally).

On Figure 3, incidental note is made of numerous uterine fibroids represented by a low signal that denotes calcification (long stem arrow). The largest fibroid arises from the left fundal region (curved arrow).

Also note the ease with which the fallopian tube and ovary on the right have been visualized in this particular case because of the serendipitous position of the ovary in the coronal plane (small arrow).

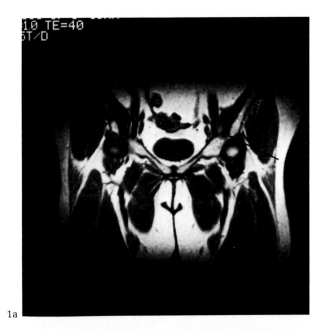

1a

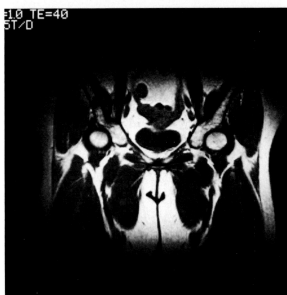

1b

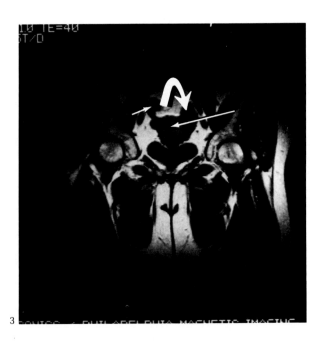

3

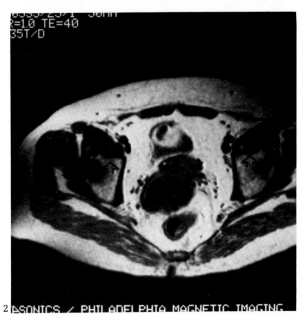

2

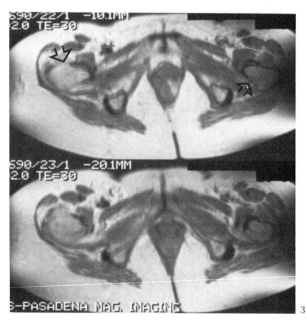

1.48 METASTASIS TO THE FEMUR

This is a 61-year-old female with known cancer and pain in the hips. Figure 1 demonstrates (curved arrows) involvement of the right femoral neck. Open arrows demonstrate typical metastatic change in the left femoral neck. There is extraosseous extension of the metastatic change on the anterior surface of the right femoral shaft at the trochanteric line (Figure 2, curved arrows) and replacement of the normal high-signal marrow in the neck and the proximal shaft on the left (Figure 2, open arrows).

Figure 3 demonstrates disruption of cortex on the right anteriorly (open arrow), as well as thinning and possible early erosion of the posterior cortex of the left femur (small open arrow).

MRI has been extremely useful in evaluating early malignant change, even with negative bone scan and negative plain x-ray films. The early detection of otherwise occult lesions facilitates more accurate staging, as well as assessment and treatment of focal bone pain unexplained by more convential workup.

This case is through the courtesy of Dr. R. S. Arora and Dr. Rodolfo A. Lopez of Pasadena Magnetic Imaging.

1.49 DERMOID OF THE SOFT TISSUES OF THE KNEE

This is a 27-year-old male. Figure 1 demonstrates a discrete small, rounded lesion. The small arrows point to the muscle from which this lesion appears to arise. The borders are very sharp and the signal is high, suggesting a fatty-type content.

Figures 2 and 3 demonstrate an even higher signal than fat demonstrated on the axial T1- and T2-weighted images (arrows).

This signal behavior is consistent with a dermoid and its contents. Also note the ease of excluding any other muscle involvement by this lesion. MRI also demonstrated the fascial planes of the thigh nicely (small arrows). This distal femoral vein and artery can also be easily identified. The vein sits slightly behind the artery and is larger, with a higher signal. In this case, the increase in signal reflects the direction of blood flow rather than concern for a thrombosis.

Soft tissue masses such as the one demonstrated here can be beautifully mapped out before surgical excision. Focal attachments to local structures such as surrounding bone and muscle can also be evaluated.

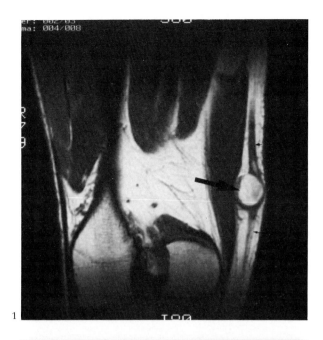

1

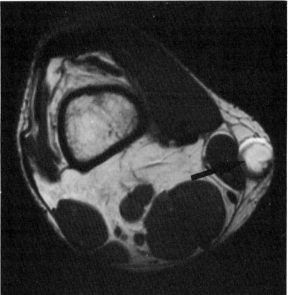

2

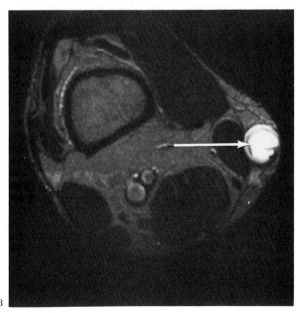

3

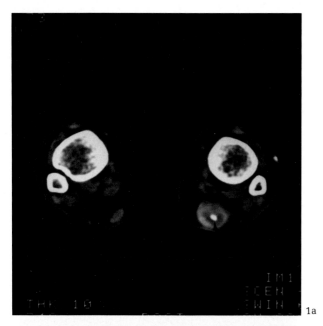

1a

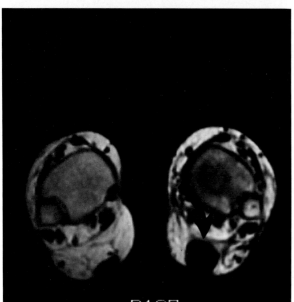

1b

1.50 HEMANGIOMA OF THE ACHILLES TENDON

This case of a 73-year-old female compares the different modalities used to assess a soft tissue abnormality.

Figure 1a is a CT cut through the abnormally thickened tendon, with a rounded calcification believed to represent a phlebolith. Figure 1b is an axial cut through the same level; the enlarged tendon is again recognized (curved arrow). The tendons and bone detail are more impressive on the MRI scan.

Figure 2a is a sagittal MRI cut through the enlarged Achilles tendon; because of the low signal intensity of the predominantly tendinous structure, the small calcifications are not well seen. Figure 2b is a plain lateral film that does demonstrate the calcified structures and confirms the suspicion, raised by the CT scan, that these represent phleboliths. The phleboliths, in turn, are highly consistent with a benign mass such as a hemangioma.

Figure 3a demonstrates the T1 appearance in the coronal plane. Figure 3b demonstrates the tendon with increased signal within it. This reflects venous flow, which is better appreciated on the T2-weighted image.

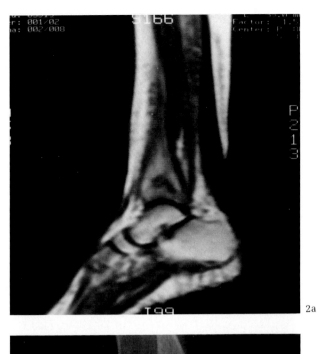

2a

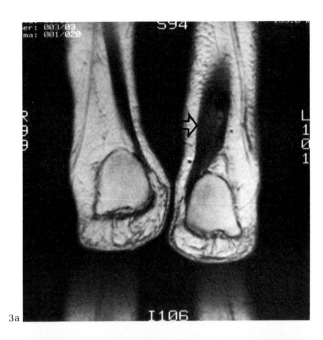

3a

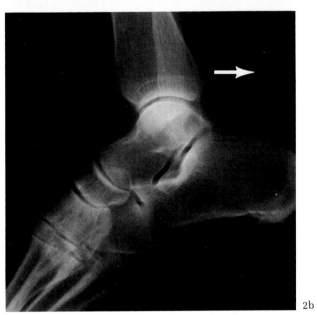

2b

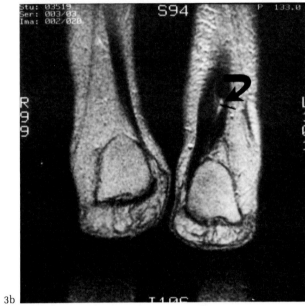

3b

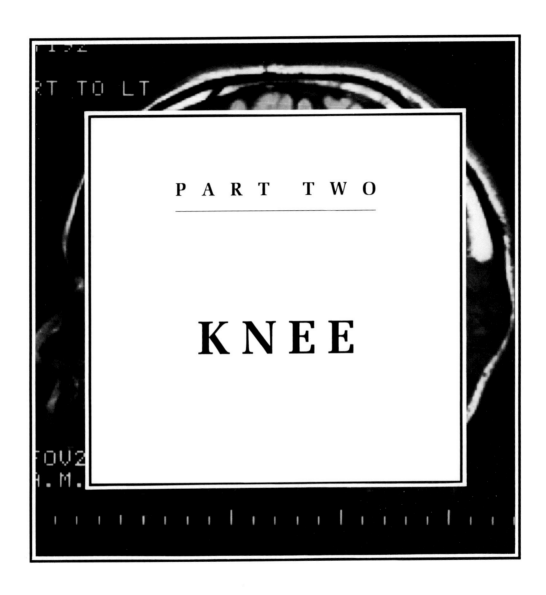

PART TWO

KNEE

2.1 FOCAL CHONDROMALACIA OF THE PATELLA

Figure 1 (arrows) demonstrates thinning of the articular cartilage, as well as subchondral change in the patellar bone revealing an area of lateral chondromalacia. The middle and medial portions of the patellar cartilage are maintained. The patient did complain of pain, which lateralized to the side of the findings. Figure 2 also demonstrates the subchondral changes, and the two small arrows show a slight break in the normal low-signal subcortical bone, again indicating the changes deep to the now damaged patellar cartilage. Figure 3 is a sagittal representation of this irregularity within the patella, demonstrating some scalloping, as well as interruption of the subchondral cortical bone (arrow).

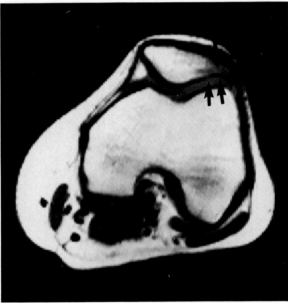

1

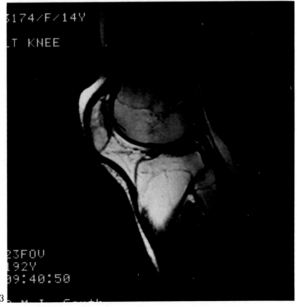

2

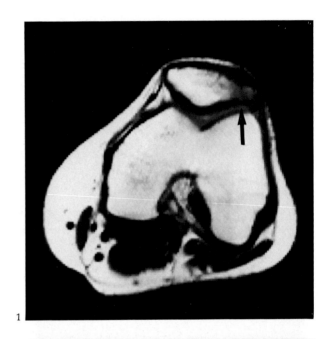

3

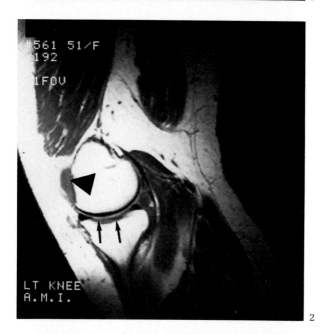

1

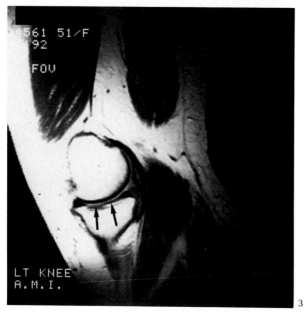

2

3

2.2 MEDIAL MENISCUS BUCKET HANDLE TEAR

Figures 1 to 4 are contiguous sagittal images through the medial meniscus demonstrating persistent widening rather than a decrease in the space between the anterior and posterior horns. The abnormal persistence of widening suggests absence of part of the peripheral portion of the meniscus, which is consistent with a large bucket handle tear. On Figure 5 (coronal image) there is evidence of a blunted, deformed medial meniscus rather than the normal well-outlined, dark triangle representing the meniscus.

Figures 1 and 2 (arrowhead) demonstrate a small effusion.

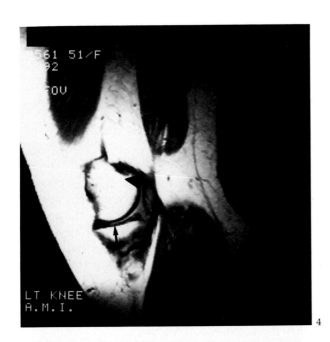

4

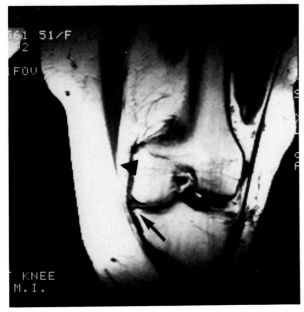

5

2.3 DIFFUSE DEGENERATIVE CHANGE WITHIN THE MEDIAL MENISCUS

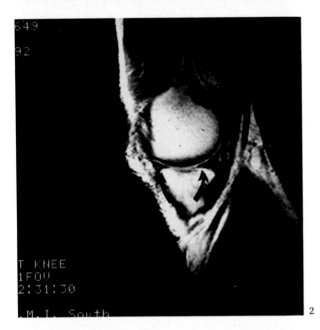

1

The medial meniscus appears intact in its outer contour; however, there is a central increase in signal. In the painful knee, this represents a degenerative change within the substance of the meniscus and suggests a predisposition to possible tearing injury. Figure 1 demonstrates the increase in signal of the medial meniscus (arrows). Note that the lateral meniscus also shows a slight increase in signal, although it is not as intense (curved arrow).

Figures 2 and 3 demonstrate increased signal within the anterior and posterior horns, again reflecting degenerative change within the substance of the meniscus.

Note the Baker's cyst in Figure 3, which is further proof of internal derangement within the knee joint.

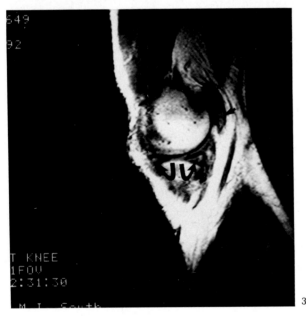

2

3

2.4 STATUS AFTER MEDIAL MENISCECTOMY

Figure 1a demonstrates a lateral meniscus (arrowheads) and absence of the medial meniscus (curved arrow). Figure 1b is a slightly more posterior coronal image demonstrating the same findings. Note the alteration of the signal of the femoral condyle medially, suggestive of some early sclerotic change representing a degenerative reaction in the medial knee compartment.

Figures 2 and 3 are contiguous sagittal images moving lateral, again demonstrating absence of a visualized meniscus in the medial knee compartment. This patient had a prior meniscectomy.

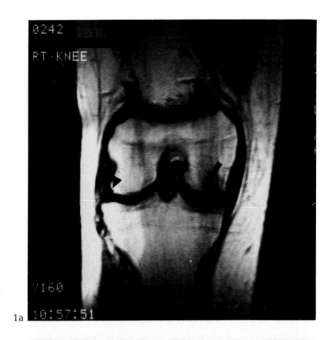

1a

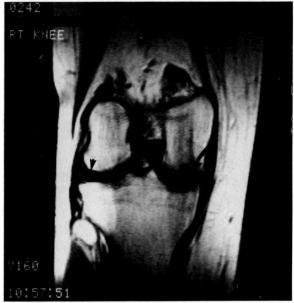

1b

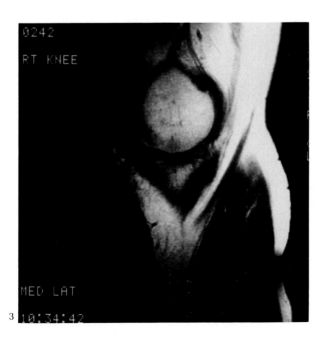

3

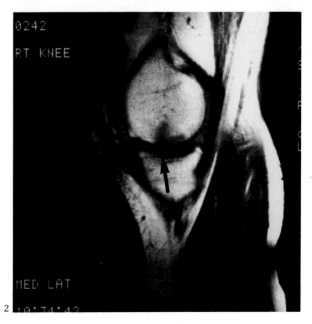

2

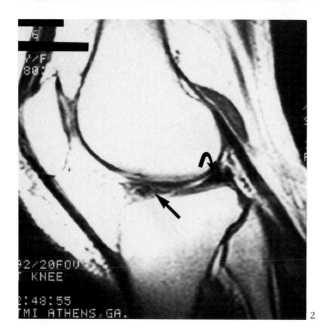

2.5 EXTENSIVE LATERAL MENISCAL DAMAGE WITH GEODE

Figures 1 and 2 are sagittal cuts through the lateral meniscus demonstrating the normal posterior horn (curved arrow) and the grossly abnormal anterior horn (straight arrows). Note the loss of normal low signal, as well as enlargement of the anterior horn. There is also a diffuse increased signal running through the meniscal structure consistent with complex tearing. This represents a combination of horizontal and vertical tearing of the meniscus.

Figure 3 demonstrates, in a coronal image, the lateral meniscus, again torn.

Incidental note is made of a tiny geode that represents a subchondral cyst extending from the medial portion of the lateral knee compartment. Figure 4 is a sagittal representation of this geode. The geode represents a break in the cartilage that allows fluid to extend into the subchondral bone and cause focal expansion.

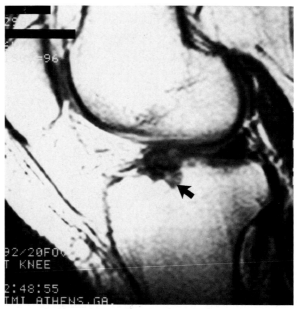

2.6 MEDIAL MENISCUS BUCKET HANDLE TEAR

Figures 1a and 1b demonstrate a blunted, deformed medial meniscus with increased signal centrally (arrows).

Figure 2 demonstrates the widened appearance of the anterior and posterior horns, with poor visualization of any peripheral meniscus. Also note the blunted appearance of the horns.

Figure 3 suggests the presence, in the slightly more lateral sagittal cut, of a small free fragment of the bucket handle-type tear (curved arrow).

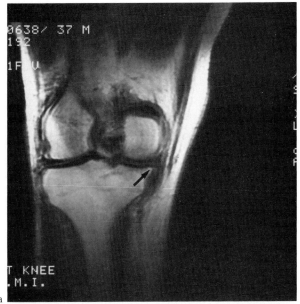

1a

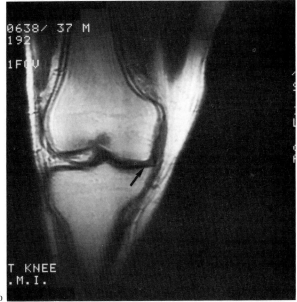

1b

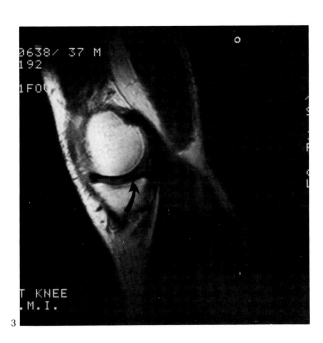

3

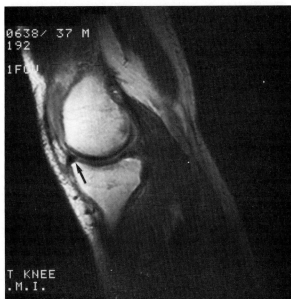

2

2.7 MEDIAL MENISCAL TEAR

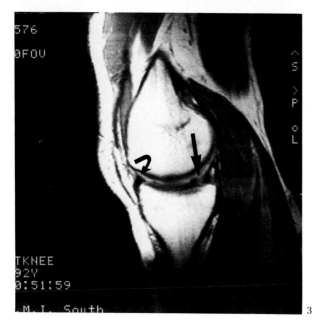

Figure 1 is a nice demonstration of the blunting of the medial meniscus consistent with a tear through its peripheral edge. Figure 2 demonstrates a distorted, torn posterior horn, and Figure 3 demonstrates additional deformity of this horn. The open arrows point to the anterior horns for comparison with the more normal appearance of the meniscus anteriorly.

Figure 1 also demonstrates nicely, in the coronal plane, the horizontal normal appearance of the posterior cruciate ligament, which is medial (arrow); adjacent to it is the anterior cruciate ligament (open arrow).

2.8 HEMOARTHROSIS

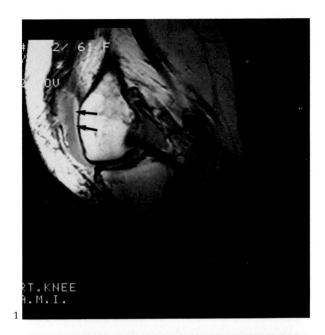

The simple joint effusion can be easily recognized with MRI, particularly when one inspects the lateral recesses and the suprapatellar bursa. It is also helpful to note when the effusion contains more than one component. Fatty material will float or rise to the most superior portion of the knee joint. Blood will separate into levels, with the effusion demonstrating a fluid-fluid level. Note on Figure 1 the high signal intensity seen with the hematocrit, which has separated from the serum, and simple effusion.

When the multiple-component effusion is demonstrated, the search for underlying bone fracture and possible ligament disruption should be thorough.

Figures 2 and 3 demonstrate the effusion on the lateral aspect of the knee joint; the separation is slightly less well appreciated. Also note the patellar changes consistent with chondromalacia.

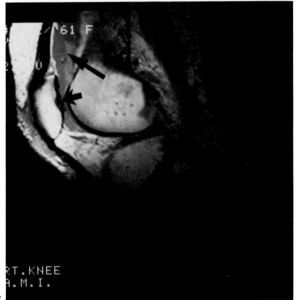

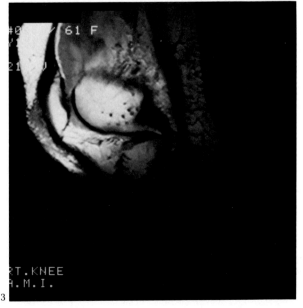

2.9 LARGE EFFUSIONS OF THE KNEE

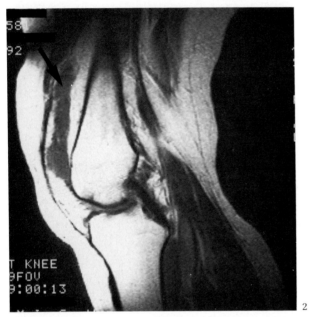

1

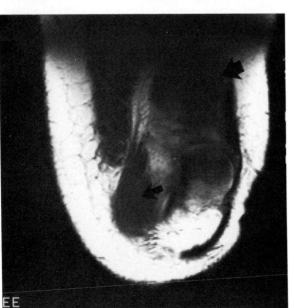

2

The large effusions demonstrate nicely where smaller pockets of fluid can be searched for in the less obviously abnormal knee joint. Note that a large amount of the effusion resides in the suprapatellar bursa when the patient is supine. Figure 1 demonstrates this finding (arrows). Also note that the posterior cruciate ligament is normal in appearance. Sometimes large effusions can cause signal averaging with normal structures, making recognition of cruciate tears more difficult.

Note too that the suprapatellar bursa extends superiorly along the length of the femur. Often the only trace of joint fluid seen will be within this portion of the supine knee joint (large arrow, Figure 2).

Figure 3 demonstrates the appearance of the fluid in the coronal plane. In the predominantly T1-weighted image, the fluid has a low signal and is smooth in appearance (arrows). The effusion, if large enough, will also surround the patella.

3

2.10 FAT/BLOOD EFFUSION OF THE KNEE JOINT

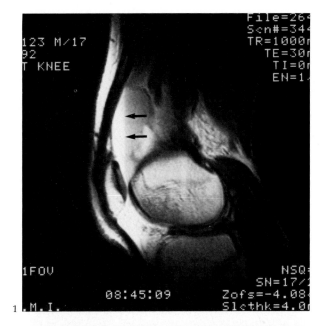

This effusion is the reverse of the bloody effusion in that the higher-signal contents are now superior to the fluid. This is consistent with the presence of fatty material within the joint effusion. Figure 1 demonstrates the fluid-fat level (arrows).

Figure 2a is a more medial cut from this same series of sagittal images, but the level can be redefined easily.

Figure 3 demonstrates the effusion surrounding the patella on a more anterior coronal image (arrows). Note that the fluid has a higher signal than the simple effusion. This suggests the presence of blood within the effusion.

This particular case shows the anterior cruciate course. The normal anterior cruciate is visualized as a dark, continuous band that arises from the tibial spine and projects posteriorly to insert behind the femur (Figure 2b). In this particular case, the effusion, because of its slightly higher signal, helps to outline and define the structure. Simple effusions, because of their low signal, can blend with and even obscure the ligament.

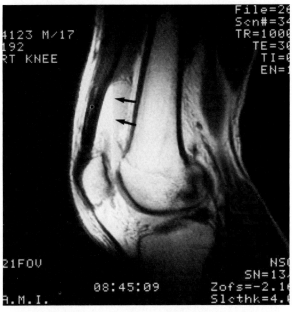

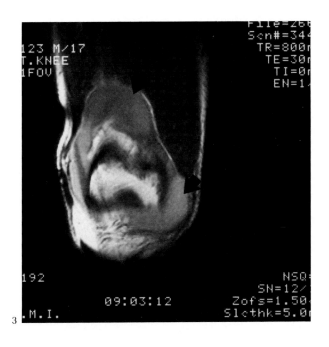

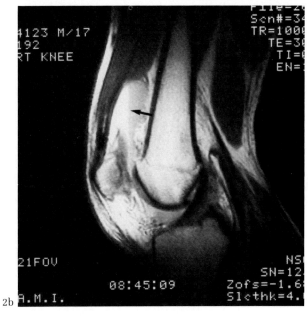

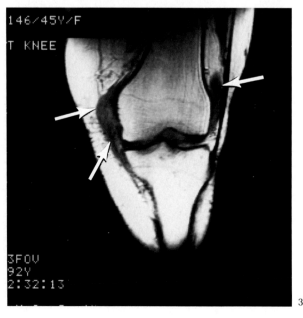

2.11 MEDIAL COLLATERAL LIGAMENT DAMAGE

The medial collateral ligament is shown by a continuous thin band of low signal along the medial aspect of the knee. Figure 1 demonstrates the torn appearance of the ligament, as well as the fluid that surrounds the ligament. Additionally, the soft tissues around the ligament should be homogeneous and should show a high signal. Smaller strains and tears can be detected not by direct visualization of the torn ligament but by the soft tissue edema.

Figure 2 again shows the irregular appearance of the ligament. Note that an effusion can distend the collateral ligament but that the effusion has a smooth border. Also, the size of the effusion can be correlated with the sagittal and axial images. Focal irregular pockets to the side of the knee surrounding the ligament usually reflect damage to the ligament.

Figure 3 is an even more anterior coronal cut from this series, showing the disrupted appearance of the ligament once again.

2.12 PATELLAR TENDON DISRUPTION

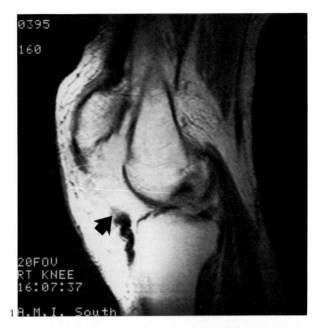

Severe trauma can disrupt even the patellar ligament. Figure 1 demonstrates, in the sagittal plane, the torn tendon (arrow). The attachment to the tibia is preserved, but the entire tendon midsustance has been torn. Figure 2 is another of the coronal images in the set, again confirming that the whole tendon has been torn. Also note that the effusion, aside from being quite large, is higher in signal than a simple effusion and is consistent with the presence of a hemorrhagic component.

The sagittal plane is best for examining the patellar tendon. The normal tendon is discrete and low signal in appearance.

Note the intact anterior cruciate ligament in Figure 2. It is slightly stretched but intact.

Figure 3a demonstrates a coronal cut through the disrupted ligament (arrow). Figure 3b is an axial cut through the joint. Note both the large effusion and the medial deviation of the now untethered patellar bone.

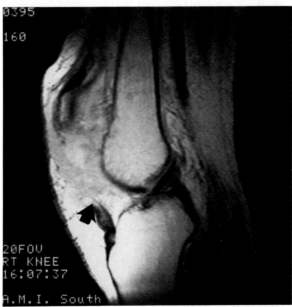

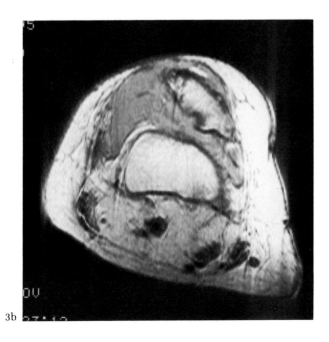

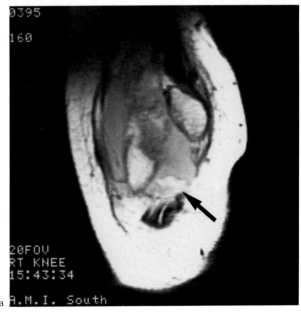

2.13 ANTERIOR CRUCIATE TEAR

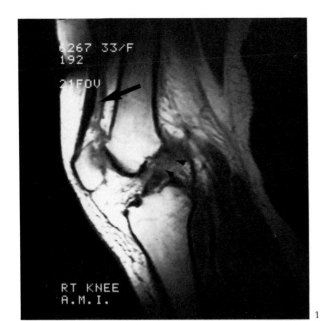

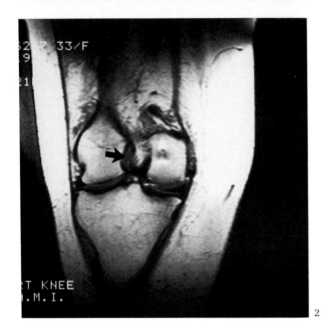

The anterior cruciate ligament is perhaps the hardest of the ligaments to image correctly. We now flex and slightly rotate the knee to put the anterior ligament into a more orthogonal plane for imaging purposes. It is also crucial to examine the knee in at least two planes, and preferably in three planes. A repeat sagittal plane attempt with slight further rotation may be needed if the anterior cruciate ligament is not well seen on the routine images. The anterior cruciate ligament inserts on the tibial spine and projects posteriorly to insert along the back of the distal femur. Small effusions can sometimes hide the anterior cruciate ligament and may simulate a tear.

Figure 1 demonstrates the torn anterior cruciate. Note that there is also an effusion and that corroboration with Figure 2, a coronal image, is a valuable check (arrow). Note the higher signal in the region of the normal course of an anterior cruciate versus the low-signal appearance of a posterior cruciate (arrow).

2.14 FIBULAR COLLATERAL LIGAMENT TEAR

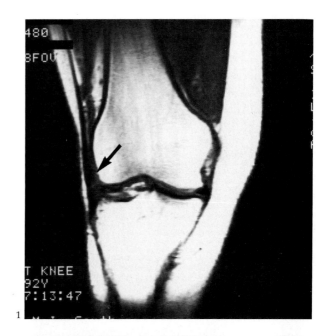

The collateral ligaments, although easily evaluated clinically, can be visualized on MRI of the knee and hence should always be inspected.

The medial or tibial collateral is a part of the knee capsule and should be a continuous dark band extending alongside the knee joint.

The fibular or lateral ligament is not quite an intimate part of the capsule, but it still should maintain a dark image representing a low signal on the T1-weighted image.

Figure 1 demonstrates the disrupted fibular ligament and the surrounding edema (arrow). Figure 2 demonstrates the disruption on a more posterior cut through the coronal images.

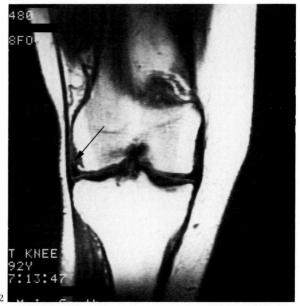

Figure 3 is a sagittal cut through this same knee that shows the presence of an effusion and a posterior horn tear (arrow). Note that often the fibular head is included in the sagittal cuts (arrowhead) and can be a helpful guide to orientation. Remember that the MRI images are processed on a computer, and human error can cause mislabeling. Orientation can also be suspect in some magnets without a dedicated knee coil. Technologists can make excellent images with the head coil or cervical spine-coil, but these reverse the normal orientation built into the software.

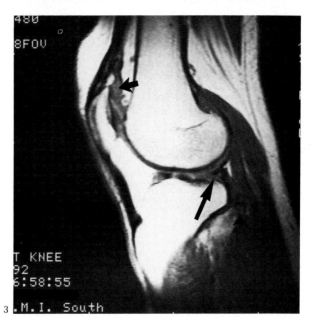

2.15 POSTERIOR CRUCIATE LIGAMENT TEAR

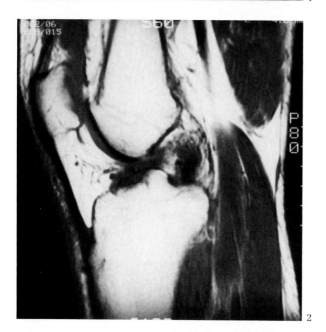

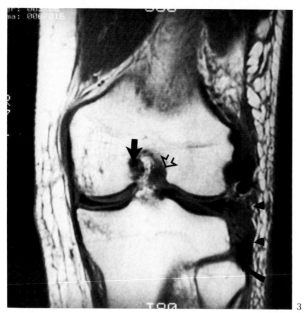

Figure 1 demonstrates a lack of visualization of the normal posterior ligament (arrow). In addition, a large effusion is present (arrowheads).

Figure 2 is another image from the same sagittal series. All images in the sagittal plane failed to visualize the posterior ligament.

The posterior ligament is easily appreciated even on scout images, when intact. It is large and maintains a low signal throughout its structure.

Figure 3 is a coronal image of the knee (the open arrow points to the area where the anterior cruciate ligament should be). Note the loss of normal low signal, as seen with the posterior cruciate ligament (large solid arrow).

2.16 FIBULAR COLLATERAL LIGAMENT TEAR

This is a marked disruption of the fibular or lateral collateral ligament. Figure 1 demonstrates a large amount of fluid that represents edema and hemorrhage in the lateral soft tissue adjacent to the knee. There is no evidence of a dark band-like structure that could represent the ligament. The curved arrows on both Figures 1 and 2 point to what may be the remains of a ligament within the traumatic mass of soft tissue.

Note also that the normally high-signal subcutaneous fat is now streaky in appearance, consistent with diffuse edema surrounding the damaged ligament.

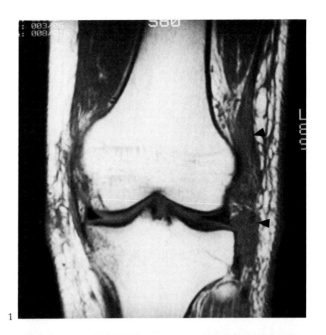

1

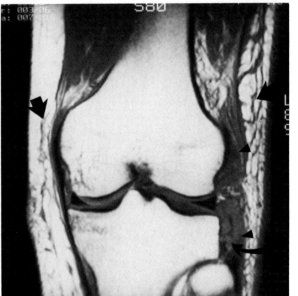

2

2.17 MEDIAL COLLATERAL LIGAMENT TEAR

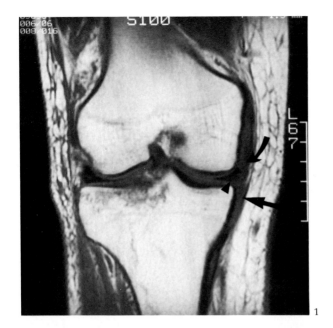

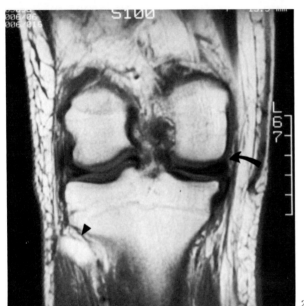

Figure 1 (curved arrows) demonstrates the disrupted appearance of the medial or tibial collateral ligament. There is also high signal in the lateral portion of the medial meniscus, suggesting that the collateral ligament has been torn from the meniscus (arrowhead). A nonspecific area of intermediate signal replaces the high signal of the surrounding fat, and there is loss of the normal thin band of low signal that should be the medial collateral ligament.

Figure 2 is a more posterior coronal cut in the same series. The findings are again appreciated (curved arrow). Note that the fibular head can also be seen on this image, allowing confirmation of the medial or lateral location of the abnormality.

2.18 NORMAL PATELLAR TENDON

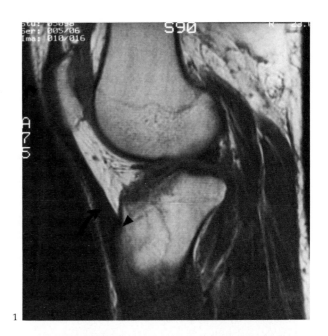

The normal tendon can be seen as a low-signal structure that arises from the inferior pole of the patellar bone to insert onto the tibial tuberosity (Figure 1, arrowhead). Figure 2 demonstrates nicely the normal appearance of the patellar tendon. Also note that the infrapatellar fat pad (small arrows) is well evaluated in the sagittal plane.

The sagittal plane is most helpful for evaluation of the tendon, and it should be examined as a routine part of the MRI exam of the knee.

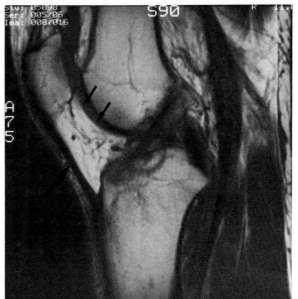

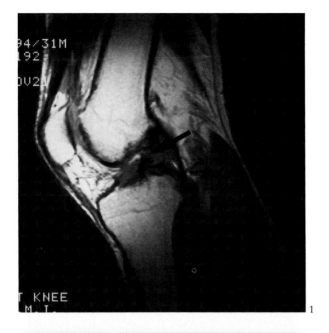

1

2.19 ANTERIOR CRUCIATE TEAR

In this case, the inferior segment of the ligament is still attached and is visualized on Figure 1 (curved arrow). Figures 2a and 2b demonstrate, on the coronal images, the appearance of the torn cruciate ligament (long-stem arrows). This appearance can be compared to that of the intact posterior ligament seen on Figure 3 (arrowhead).

Also note the course of the attached fragment. It appears to be floating rather than having the straight, tethered look of an uninterrupted ligament.

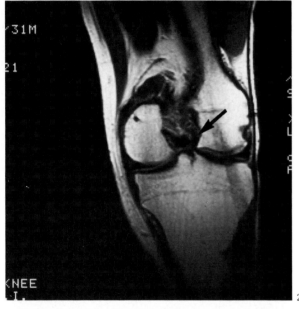

2a

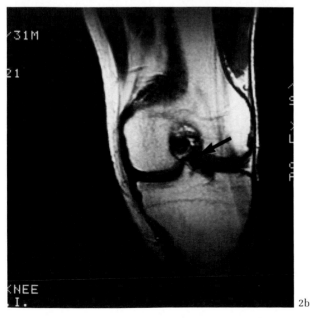

2b

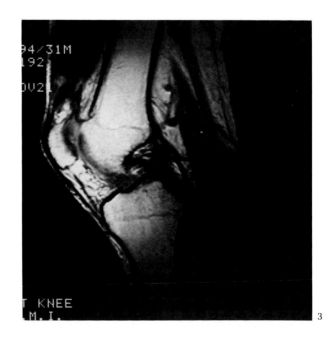

3

86

2.20 ANTERIOR LIGAMENT TEAR WITH LARGE EFFUSION

Figure 1 is a sagittal cut through the area of the anterior cruciate ligament. The open arrows denote the area where the ligament should be visualized. A large effusion is indicated by a curved arrow.

With a large effusion, such as seen here, the sagittal view requires confirmation by inspection of the coronal views.

Figures 2 and 3 demonstrate the absence of the anterior cruciate ligament (large arrows). Compare this to the dark appearance or low signal of the posterior cruciate ligament seen in this same plane (arrowheads).

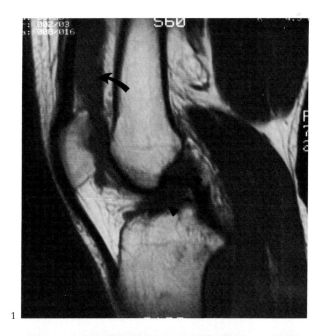

1

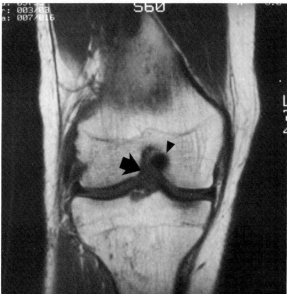

2

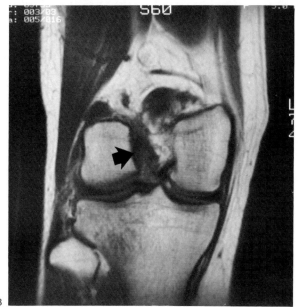

3

2.21 MEDIAL MENISCAL CYST

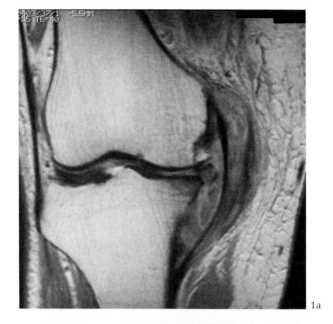

1a

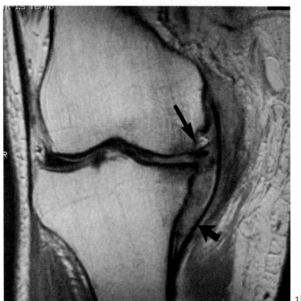

1b

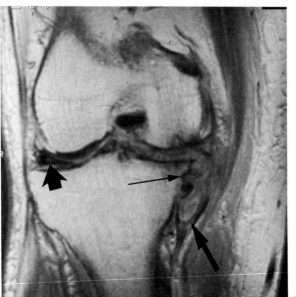

2

Figures 1a and 1b demonstrate a large tumoral-looking structure arising from the medial meniscus (arrowheads). The curved arrow shows the nearly totally destroyed medial meniscus from which the cyst has arisen. Figure 2 is slightly more posterior in the coronal orientation and shows the large size of the cyst (arrow). Also note that there is some erosion of the bone associated with this cyst. Again note that the meniscus has been largely destroyed. The lateral meniscus is present (large arrow). One theory of cyst development relates to tears in the meniscus that permit fluid to become trapped in the meniscus, allowing cyst formation to occur. This case supports this theory of cyst development.

Figures 3a and 3b demonstrate the appearance of the cyst in the sagittal plane. Note the almost tumoral appearance of the cyst. Curved arrows demonstrate the loss of normal meniscus morphology. The tumoral appearance was such that the patient underwent a biopsy of this mass. Retrospectively, however, we would not expect a tumor to destroy the meniscus.

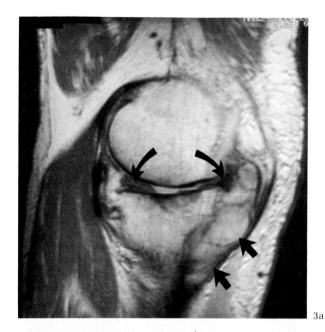

3a

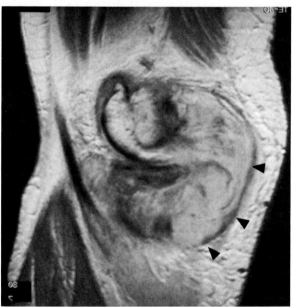

3b

89

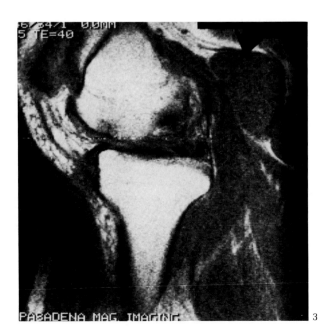

2.22 LARGE BAKER'S CYST OR POPLITEAL CYST

Figure 1 demonstrates a large popliteal cyst, with the technique of a T2-weighted image causing an increased signal from the joint fluid (arrow). There is also a small amount of fluid within the joint capsule for comparison (small arrow).

These cysts represent bursal collections of fluid that can occur around the knee joint. The underlying cause of these cysts is related to the trauma or arthritis. Communication with the cyst can be seen in about half of the cysts. Figures 2a and 2b are axial cuts through the joint, and the curved arrow demonstrates the communication of the capsule with the cyst. The cyst is outlined by arrowheads.

Figure 3 is a T1-weighted image of the cyst in the sagittal plane. Note that the signal is similar to that seen in the muscle (arrow).

These studies are usually requested for the workup of a palpable mass posterior to the knee. Arthrography does not demonstrate all of these cysts, and their detection with MRI is straightforward.

This case is through the courtesy of Dr. Hal Boone and Dr. J.R. Herrara of Pasadena Magnetic Imaging.

90

2.23 FREE FRAGMENT SECONDARY TO MENISCAL TEAR

Figures 1a and 1b demonstrate visualization of a fragment lying in the midknee compartment separate from the medial meniscus (large arrows).

Figure 2 is a sagittal cut demonstrating the disrupted, abnormal appearance of the anterior horn, and Figure 3 is a coronal image demonstrating the partially blunt free edge of the medial meniscus where the tear has occurred. In visualization of a free fragment, one must be careful that averaging of the cortex of the femoral condyle is not read as representing free fragment. On Figures 1a and 1b, the curved arrows demonstrate the normal appearance of the femoral cortical line.

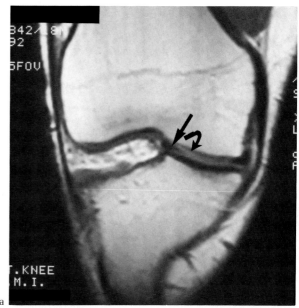

1a

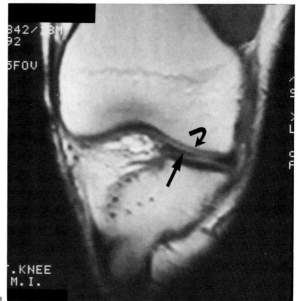

1b

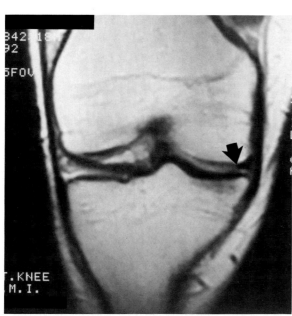

3

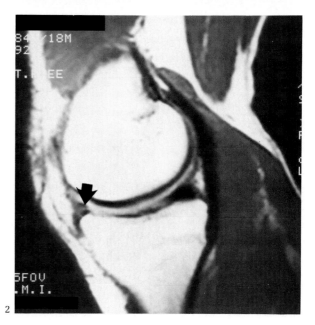

2

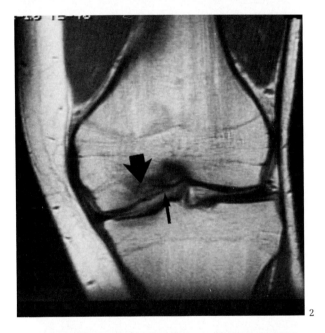

1

A discrete area of slightly decreased signal in the medial aspect of the lateral femoral condyle in a 17-year-old male is identified on coronal Figures 1 and 2. There is also disruption of the normal low signal from the cortical bone (small arrows). Figures 3a and 3b demonstrate, in the sagittal plane, the appearance of this area of decreased signal (large arrow), and small arrows again designate the disruption of the normal low-signal cortical line. Findings are consistent with osteochondrosis dissecans. The location is typical, and the patient's age and clinical presentation are also quite typical of this finding.

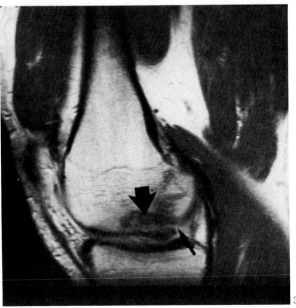

2

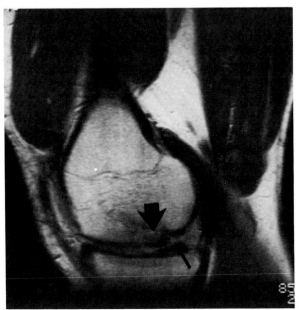

3a

3b

2.25 INTRA-ARTICULAR LOOSE BODY

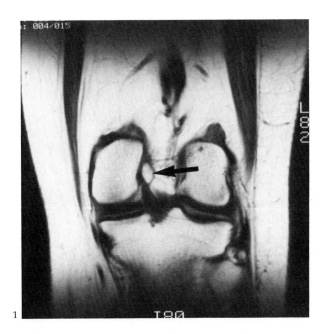

Figure 1 demonstrates, in the coronal image, a large intra-articular body. Despite the size of the image and the clinical history, which are consistent with a loose body, the sagittal images through this area, represented by Figures 2 and 3, fail to confirm the presence of this body, which was believed to be present both on clinical grounds and on the basis of the coronal images.

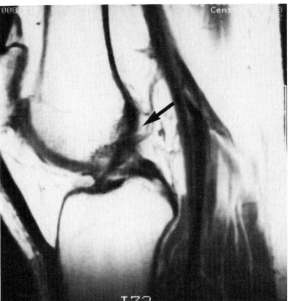

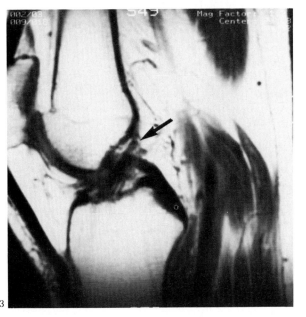

2.26 OSTEOCHONDRITIS DISSECANS

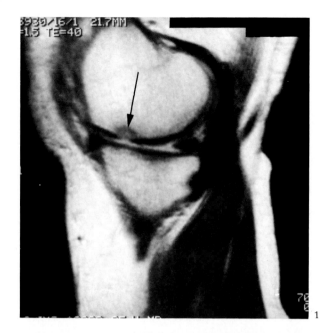

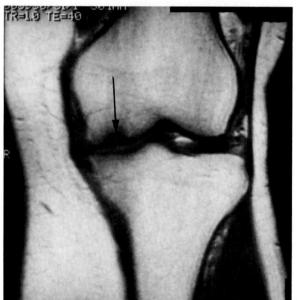

This typical defect in the subchondral region of the femoral condyle is identified on Figure 1 in the sagittal cut (long-stemmed arrow). The appearance of the defect is again confirmed in the coronal cuts through this same area (Figure 2, long-stemmed arrow). Findings are consistent with osteochondritis dissecans. This is a somewhat unusual lesion for a patient of this age and sex (a 61-year-old female). It is most often seen in children and in young adults, usually male.

This case is through the courtesy of Dr. Robert Chiteman of Maryland Magnetic Imaging.

2.27 MILD TO MODERATE CHANGES OF CHONDROMALACIA

This images are from the same sagittal series, moving medial to lateral. Figure 1 demonstrates the presence of an effusion with a curved arrow. No other meniscal or ligament tear or bony abnormalities were seen, and painful knee that is particularly common in young adults is most likely secondary to damage to the patellar cartilage or chondromalacia. The cartilaginous covering of the femoral condyle anteriorly is partially visualized with the open arrow in Figure 1. The patellar cartilage is not as well appreciated, and there is concern about a defect that extends into the subchondral bone (large arrow). Figure 2 is a more lateral sagittal cut. The curved arrow again points to the defect within the subchondral bone that suggests the presence of a tear and damage to the overlying patellar cartilage. Figure 3 is an even more lateral cut. The open arrow again points to the normal intact island cartilage covering the femoral condyle. The curved arrow demonstrates some early decreased signal in the subchondral bone of the patella, further indirect evidence for the presence of chondromalacia.

We have added axial imaging of the patellar cartilage as a routine part of our knee investigation after earlier experience and underevaluation of the patellar cartilage based on the sagittal views alone.

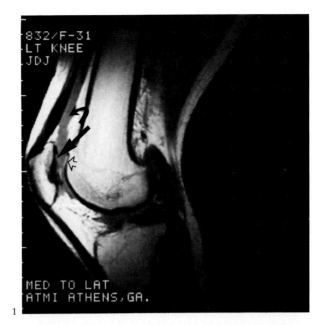

1

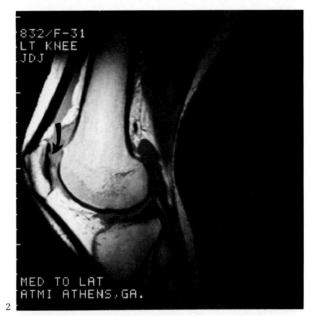

2

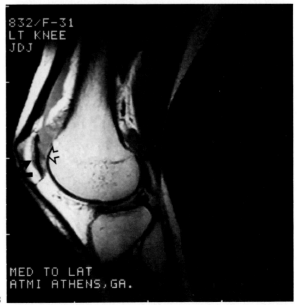

3

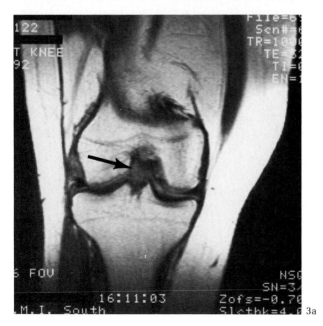

2.28 LARGE ANTERIOR CRUCIATE TEAR AND HEMATOMA

This example shows a large focus of fluid surrounding the anterior cruciate ligament. Figure 1 demonstrates the sagittal appearance of the collection in the area where the cruciate ligament should be observed (arrows).

Figures 1 and 2 demonstrate the bony attachment of the anterior cruciate to the tibial spine (curved arrows). Note that there is no effusion. The cruciate structure within the knee capsule is extrasynovial.

Figures 3a and 3b are coronal cuts through the knee demonstrating the torn ligament (arrow). Note the relationship to the posterior cruciate ligament (open arrow).

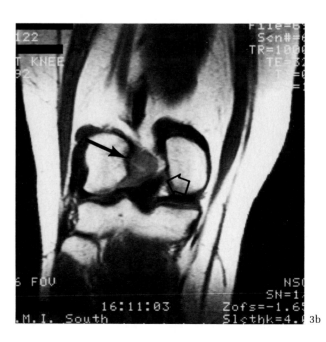

2.29 MEDIAL MENISCAL TEAR

Figure 1 is a sagittal cut through the medial meniscus that demonstrates an incomplete vertical tear through the posterior horn of the meniscus (arrow). Figure 2 is a mid- to posterior coronal cut through the knee again demonstrating the tear (arrow). Figure 3, another coronal image from the same series, again demonstrates the tear (arrow). Note the posterior cruciate is readily identified and can be useful to orient the abnormality laterally or medially.

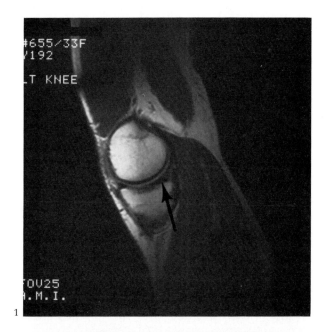

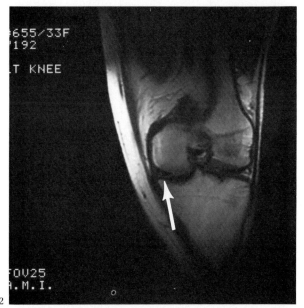

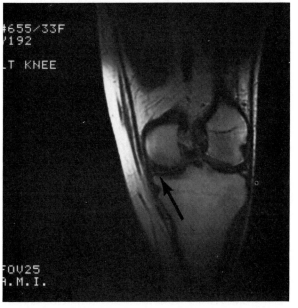

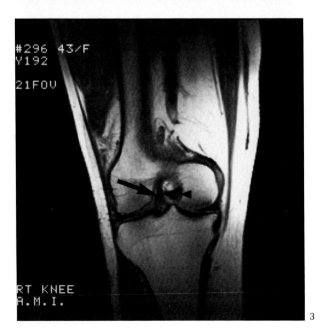

2.30 ANTERIOR CRUCIATE LIGAMENT TEAR WITH EFFUSION

Sagittal images of the knee, shown in Figures 1 and 2, fail to demonstrate the normal anterior cruciate ligament. The curved arrows show the region where the femoral portion of the ligament should be. There is also edema and a fluid collection in this region (arrowhead). Note too that a large effusion is present (short arrow).

The coronal image (Figure 3) can be useful in confirming the sagittal image finding. The anterior cruciate should be present as an almost vertical low-signal structure (long arrow). The posterior cruciate ligament in this image is horizontal and low signal in appearance (arrowhead).

There is an effusion present that can hide the anterior ligament, but the evidence on both coronal and sagittal images of a tear is strong, and suspicion should remain high.

2.31 LOOSE BODY WITHIN KNEE JOINT POSSIBLY SECONDARY TO OLD OSTEOCHONDRITIS DISSECANS

This is a 44-year-old male. Figure 1 demonstrates the free body posterior to the condyle (arrow). The open arrow indicates a defect in the posterior aspect of the condyle, suggesting that an old area of osteochondritis dissecans has allowed the bone fragment to become loose and migrate into the joint space.

Figure 2 is an axial cut demonstrating the joint mouse. Figure 3 is a coronal view also identifying the joint mouse. Synovial osteochondromatosis may also cause free small bones within the joint space; however, these are usually numerous. The central portion of the free fragment maintains the fatty marrow, allowing a high signal. Therefore, if these joint mice are large enough, they can be easily detected.

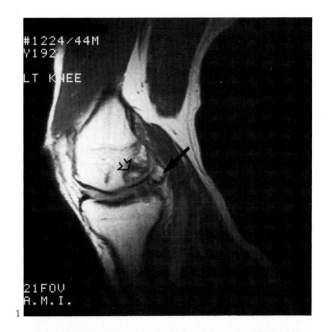

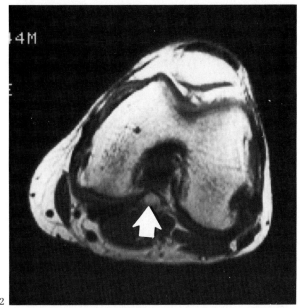

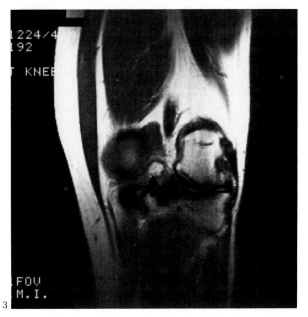

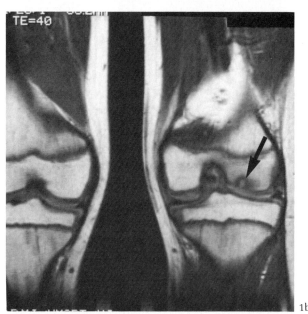
1a

This is a 12-year-old male with pain in the knee. Figures 1a and 1b demonstrate a small button of bone, separate from the femoral condyle, represented by a sclerotic, low-density rim (arrow). Compare this to the normal subchondral bone of the tibial plateau (curved arrow). Figure 2 demonstrates a more T2 proton density-weighted image, again showing maintenance of the sclerotic rim. The center button of bone maintains isointensity similar to that of the epiphyseal bone elsewhere.

Figure 3 demonstrates an incidental benign cortical defect. Osteochondritis, a disease most often affecting young males and seen in the lateral condyle, represents a small area of necrosis to the bone where the overlying cartilage has separated from the articular surface. This example involves the lateral condyle. This abnormal lesion is most commonly seen in the medial femoral condyle.

1b

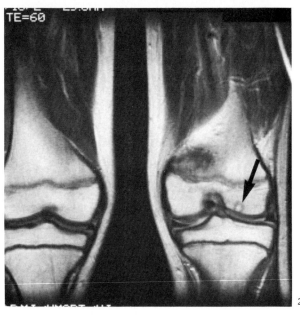
2

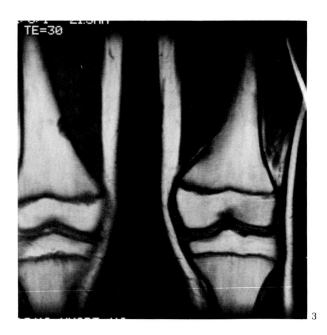
3

2.33 IMPACTION OF THE LATERAL TIBIAL PLATEAU

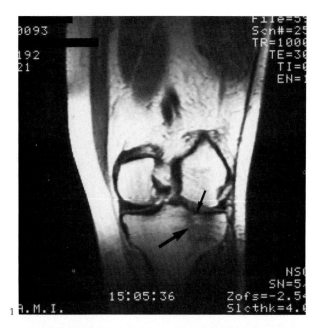

Figure 1 demonstrates mild distortion of the tibial plateau. More importantly, however, there is alteration of the normally high-signal bone marrow of the lateral tibial plateau in its subchondral aspect (large arrow). In contiguous, slightly more anterior cuts, similar findings are identified. This alteration is consistent with bone edema and suggests the presence of a possible impaction to the lateral tibial plateau. No gross dislocation is seen, and the cortex is maintained. Figure 2 is a sagittal cut through this abnormal lateral plateau, again demonstrating the altered appearance of the subchondral bone (large arrow).

On Figure 3, the curved arrow demonstrates the tibial spine and the large arrow demonstrates a portion of the anterior cruciate ligament, allowing confirmation that the coronal view and the findings refer to the lateral aspect of the tibia.

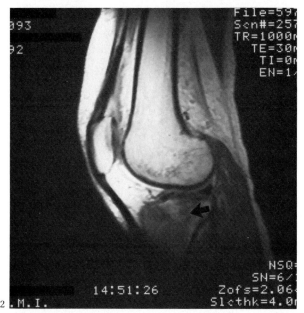

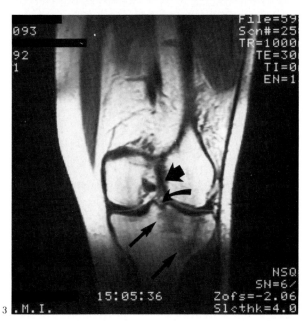

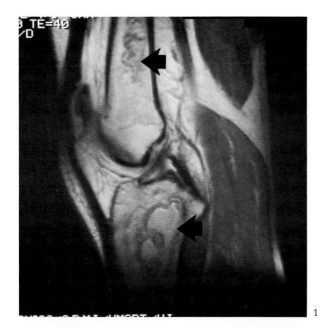

1

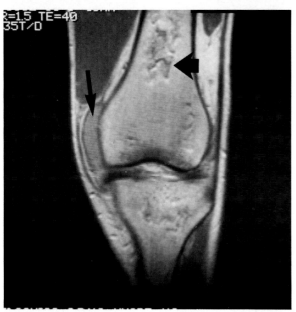

2

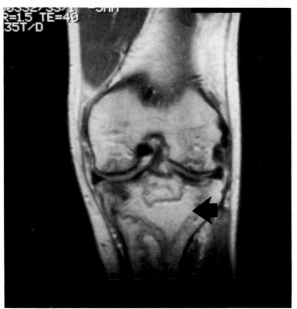

3

2.34 OSTEONECROSIS OF THE FEMUR AND TIBIA SECONDARY TO RENAL FAILURE

This patient has had a renal transplant. The MRI reveals a well-demarcated area of decreased signal involving the distal femur and tibia, which are identified on Figure 1. This is a sagittal cut through the knee.

Figure 2 demonstrates the coronal cut through the femoral bone infarct. The long-stemmed arrow demonstrates the presence of an effusion within the knee.

Figure 3 demonstrates the appearance in the coronal plane of the large bone infarct involving the tibia.

2.35 BURSAL CYST, MEDIAL KNEE

Figure 1 demonstrates a cyst arising from the medial aspect of the knee. There is a suggestion of possible communication with the more medial aspect of the knee joint slightly superior to the medial meniscus (arrow, Figure 1). Figure 2 demonstrates in the sagittal plane the appearance of the cyst. There is a small septation that may represent a small satellite cyst posterior to the large mother cyst.

Figures 3a and 3b demonstrate the axial cut through the cyst. A small joint effusion is present, allowing comparison of the joint fluid with the cyst and noting that the signal is isointense with both T1- and T2-weighted imaging. This cyst represents a collection of synovial lining with fluid accumulation. In adults these cysts usually reflect internal derangement or possibly arthritis. They are usually posterior to the knee joint, but they can occur at any location in and around the cyst. Differential concern should be raised about a possible cyst extending from the meniscus; however, no internal damage to the meniscus is seen in this particular case.

This case is courtesy of Dr. Robert Chiteman of Maryland Magnetic Imaging.

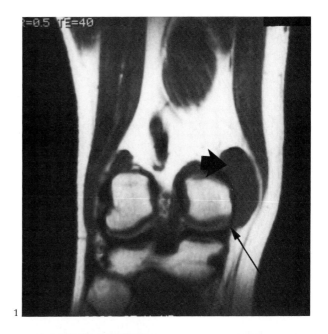

1

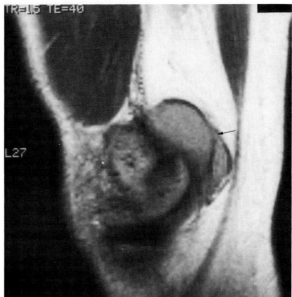

2

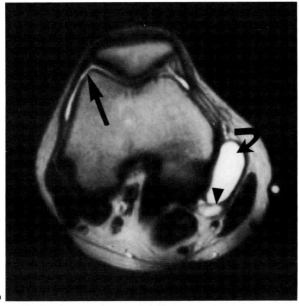

3b

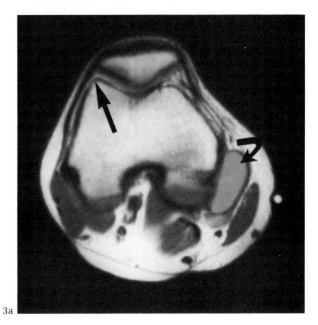

3a

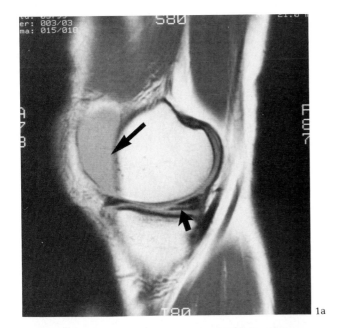

1a

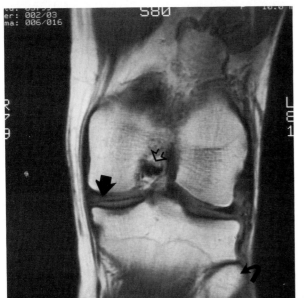

1b

2.36 HORIZONTAL MENISCAL TEAR, MEDIAL MENISCUS WITH LARGE EFFUSION

Figure 1a demonstrates nicely a horizontal tear involving the posterior horn; this is shown by the short arrow. The large arrow demonstrates an effusion within the knee joint. Figure 1b is a coronal image, with the large arrow again demonstrating the medial meniscal tear. Note that laterality can be confirmed both by visualization of the fibula (curved arrow) and by the posterior cruciate ligament (open arrow). Figure 2a is an axial cut demonstrating the effusion. Note how, in the supine position, the effusion preferentially fills into the lateral recesses of the knee joint (large arrow). Figure 2b is a sagittal cut again demonstrating where the effusion collects in the suprapatellar bursa (large arrow). This is also a nice example of a normal-appearing lateral meniscus. Note the homogeneous low signal in the lateral meniscus (open arrowheads). Compare this with Figure 1a.

Figure 3 is a coronal image demonstrating the effusion. Figure 3a shows its appearance in the suprapatellar bursa (arrow); Figure 3b, a more posterior cut, demonstrates the effusion as it appears in the lateral recess of the knee joint (long-stemmed arrows).

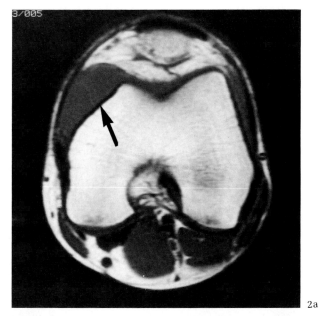

2a

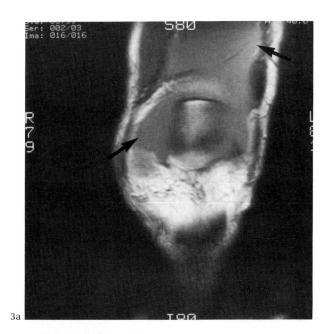

3a

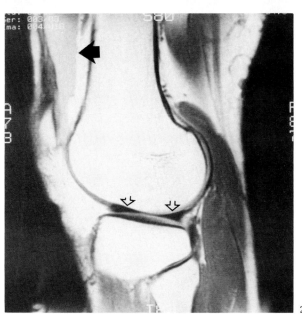

2b

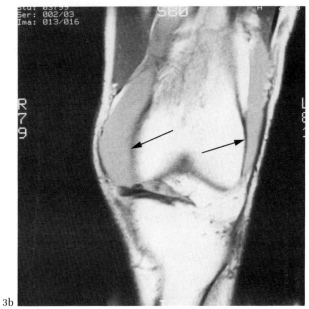

3b

2.37 HORIZONTAL TEAR WITH LARGE MEDIAL CYST

Figure 1 demonstrates increased signal through the meniscus consistent with a horizontal tear. Figure 2a demonstrates a tear communicating with the inferior surface of the meniscus (small arrow). Figures 1 and 3 also demonstrate (large arrows) a large medial degenerative cyst secondary to the tear in the meniscus that represents accumulation of fluid.

Figure 2b demonstrates a sagittal cut through the collection of the meniscal cyst; the upper and lower limits are delineated by the large arrows. Figures 2a and 2b are sagittal cuts demonstrating the horizontal tear and its communication with the inferior surface of the meniscus in the sagittal plane.

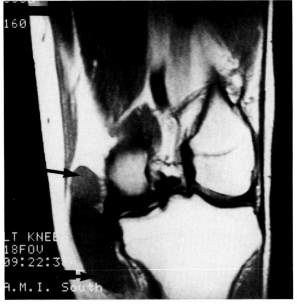

2.38 BUCKET HANDLE TEAR OF THE MEDIAL MENISCUS

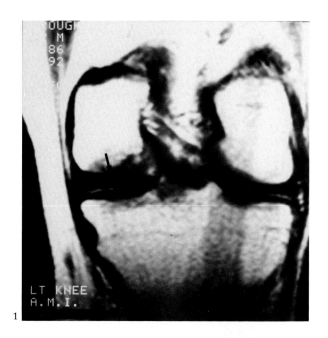

This is a contiguous series of three coronal images. Figure 1 demonstrates the intact posterior aspect of the meniscus (arrow).

The large arrow of Figure 2 demonstrates the defect through the meniscus, and the open arrow demonstrates the peripheral fragment.

Figure 3 demonstrates continuity of the tear with blunting of the still attached central portion of the meniscus (small arrow).

The long-stemmed arrow points to an area of decreased signal intensity that probably reflects the bucket handle fragment, although care must be taken not to overread the fragment, since this low signal also overlies the normal area of low signal from the cortex of the medial femoral condyle.

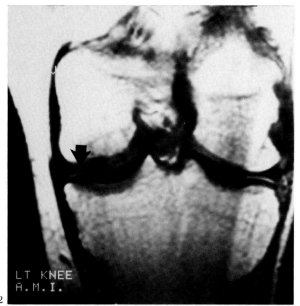

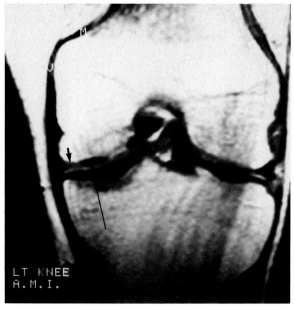

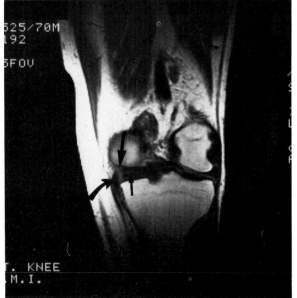

2.39 EXTENSIVE HORIZONTAL TEAR OF THE MEDIAL MENISCUS

Figure 1 demonstrates horizontal tearing and increased signal through the posterior horn of the medial meniscus. Figure 2, a slightly more medial cut, demonstrates further loss of the overall architecture of the posterior horn with increased signal. This is closer to the edge of the knee capsule, and a portion of this increased signal also reflects detachment of the tibial collateral ligament from the meniscus (Figure 3), which demonstrates (large arrow) the detachment of the meniscus with the horizontal tear (small arrow) from the tibial collateral ligament (curved arrow).

2.40 MEDIAL COLLATERAL TEAR

Figure 1, although anterior, demonstrates with a small, long-stemmed arrow the intact appearance of the inferior portion of the tibial collateral ligament as it fuses with the menisci. Superiorly, the long arrow demonstrates the directly visualized tear of the tibial collateral ligament. The pes anserinus overlying the tibial collateral ligament is still intact. The open arrow demonstrates the nonspecific collection of fluid surrounding the area of injury. Figure 2 is a slightly more anterior cut demonstrating with the curved arrow tearing of the central meniscus away from the collateral ligament. Superior to this is again the disrupted appearance of the tibial collateral ligament. The open arrow now points to what appears to be disruption of the pes anserinus. Figure 3, a slightly more anterior coronal cut, again demonstrates with the arrowhead the disruption of the meniscus from the capsule and collateral ligament, as well as a nonspecific amount of inflammatory fluid representing edema, blood, and portions of the tendinous structures (curved arrow).

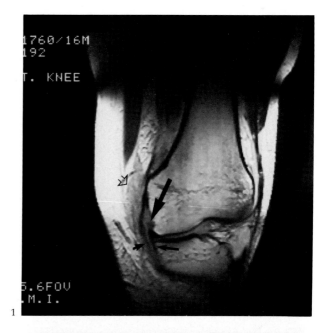

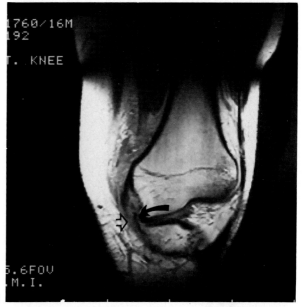

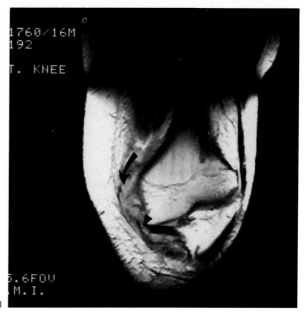

2.41 MEDIAL MENISCAL TEAR

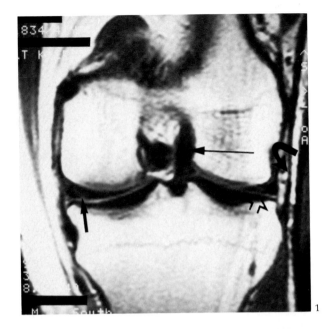

1

Figure 1 demonstrates a tear to the inferior surface of the medial meniscus (arrow). The tear is designated by increased signal in the normally low-signal meniscus. Note the increased signal in the lateral meniscus (open arrow) designating degenerative change within the meniscus laterally. Additionally, note the normal appearance of the fibular collateral ligament (curved arrow). It is important to note that this does not fuse with the meniscus, in contrast to the tibial or the medial collateral ligament.

The long-stemmed arrow points to the anterior cruciate ligament.

Figure 2a demonstrates, on a slightly more anterior cut, the continuity of the inferior cut, which extends through the central portion of the meniscus. The peripheral or thin portion of the meniscus maintains its normal contour. The long-stemmed arrow demonstrates the normal appearance of the posterior cruciate ligament. The small white arrow of Figure 2b shows an intermediate signal separating the meniscus from the overlying tendon. As the coronal cuts move anteriorly, the tibial collateral fusion with the meniscus is less well identified, and there is overlapping of the pes anserinus, which can simulate apparent detachment of the meniscus from the medial collateral ligament.

Figure 3 is a sagittal cut through the medial meniscus in its posterior horn. The small arrow demonstrates the break in the inferior surface of the medial meniscus, and the central increase in signal is also noted in the meniscus. This picture is consistent with the tear now seen in the sagittal plane. The arrowhead points to the increased signal within the posterior horn, which is abnormal.

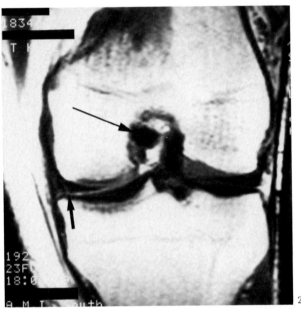

2a

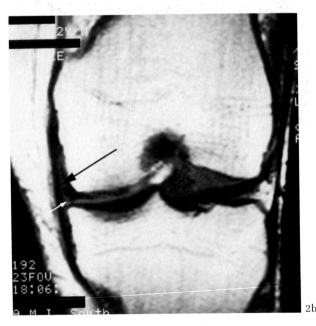

2b

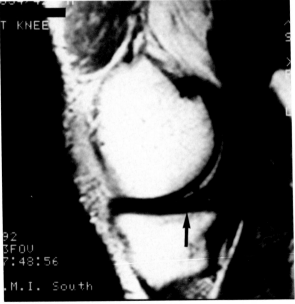

3

2.42 TIBIAL OSTEOCHONDROMA

Figure 1 demonstrates a small exostosis or osteochondroma extending from the posterior medial aspect of the proximal tibial shaft (large arrow).

A slightly more posterior cut of this lesion is seen on Figure 2 and is designated by the open arrow. Figure 3 is a sagittal cut through this same area demonstrating the intact appearance of the cortex. The lesion is demonstrated by a curved arrow. Small arrows demonstrate the cortex and its continuity with the osteochondroma.

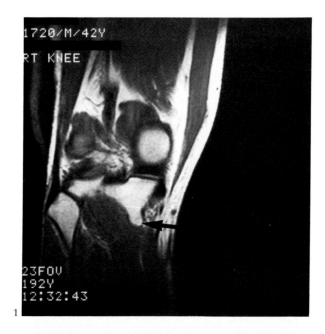

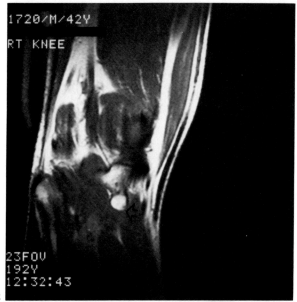

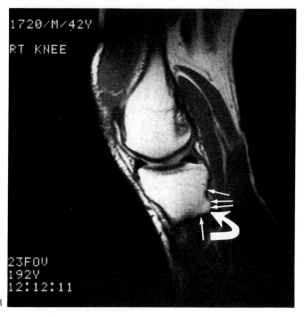

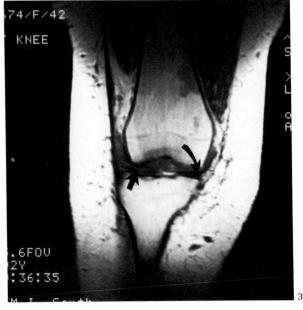

2.43 LARGE HORIZONTAL TEAR OF THE LATERAL MENISCUS WITH DEVELOPMENT OF A MENISCAL CYST

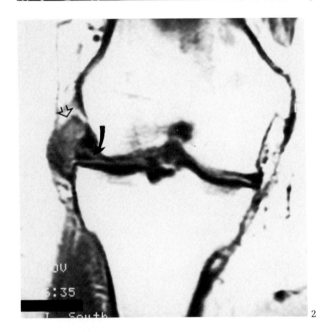

Figure 1 demonstrates a large horizontal tear through the lateral meniscus (large arrow). The small arrows demonstrate the development of a lateral meniscal cyst related to the traumatized meniscus. Figure 2 is a zoom-up view of the tear (curved arrow) and demonstrates the tear and its communication with a large meniscal cyst (open arrows).

Figure 3 is a more posterior cut contrasting the separated meniscus with a large amount of increased intermediate signal representing the tear (arrow). Compare this to the normal-appearing medial meniscus (curved arrow).

Incidental note is made of several fairly well-circumscribed areas of decreased signal within the bone marrow of the distal femur on Figure 1 (curved arrows). These most likely represent small bone infarctions; however, recent articles about bone marrow imaging also suggest a similar appearance of conversion in the adult from the yellow marrow back to a more early red marrow for the purpose of producing blood. In either case, they should not be confused with metastasis, although the differential diagnosis, particularly in patients with an appropriate clinical history, may be difficult.

2.44 MEDIAL MENISCAL TEAR WITH ASSOCIATED FRACTURE OF THE SUPERIOR PATELLA

Figure 1 demonstrates the incomplete architecture of the superior aspect of the patella. There is also an effusion (small white arrows). The open arrow designates an increase in signal and the attachment of the muscular ligament to the superior aspect of the patella, suggesting that there is soft tissue damage associated with this irregularity of the patella. A bipartite patella can be a normal variant; without the altered signal in the tendon and joint effusion, diagnosis of a fracture patella requires close clinical correlation.

Figure 2 is a slightly more medial cut again demonstrating the incomplete appearance of the superior patella, represented by the large arrow. The small white arrow again demonstrates increased signal in place of which should normally be the low signal from the ligament and bony cortex.

Figure 3 demonstrates further the defect through the superior patella.

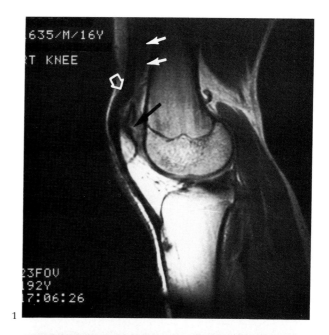

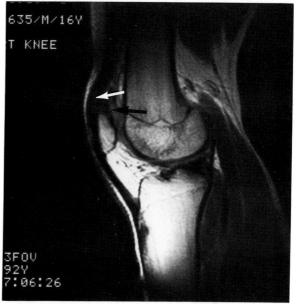

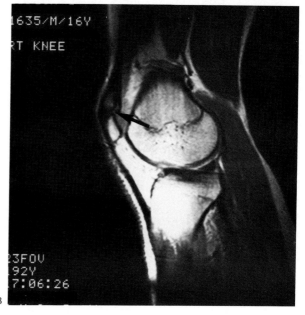

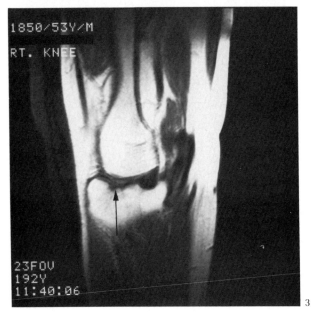

2.45 IMPACTION FRACTURE OF THE LATERAL PLATEAU

Figure 1 demonstrates decreased signal through the lateral tibial subchondral bone. There is also loss of the normal cortical detail. The menisci appear intact (short arrows). With such damage, however, close inspection of the peripheral edge of the meniscus is necessary. Associated meniscal fracture with impaction can be seen.

Figure 2 demonstrates a more lateral sagittal image. Compare the appearance of the irregular, altered cortex represented by the open arrow with that of the more anterior intact cortex (short arrow). The long arrows demonstrate decreased signal within the bone marrow representing depression of the cortex, as well as bone edema.

Figure 3 is a coronal view again confirming the irregular appearance of the tibial plateau and decreased signal in the subchondral bone, consistent with impaction fracture.

2.46 OSGOOD-SCHLATTER DISEASE

Figure 1 demonstrates slight irregularity in the tibial tuberosity of this 17-year-old male at its more lateral insertion of the patellar tendon. The low signal suggests the incomplete ossification and fusion of the tibial tubercle to the anterior tibial shaft.

Figure 2 demonstrates the slight swelling and indistinctness of the patellar tendon (small arrows). Again, areas of decreased signal in the region of the tibial tubercle and slightly inferior to it are noted. Figure 3, the most lateral cut, again demonstrates the incomplete fusion of the tibial tubercle. These findings are suggestive of Osgood-Schlatter disease, or tibial osteochondrosis of the tibial tuberosity. This diagnosis, however, requires correlation with clinical symptoms.

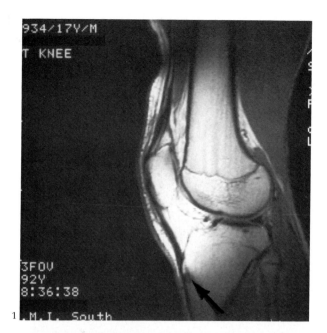

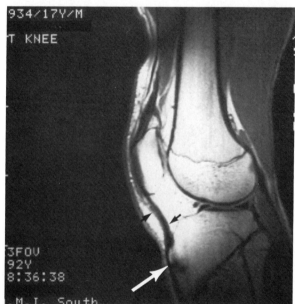

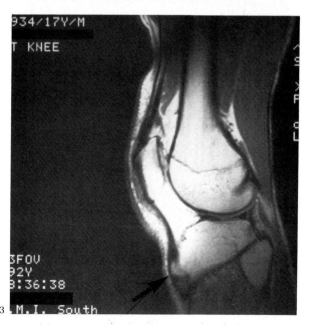

2.47 STATUS AFTER MEDIAL MENISCECTOMY

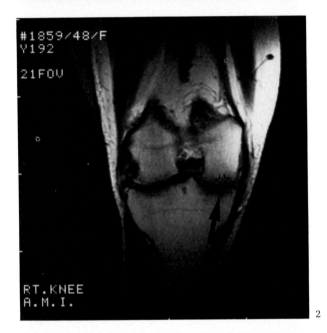

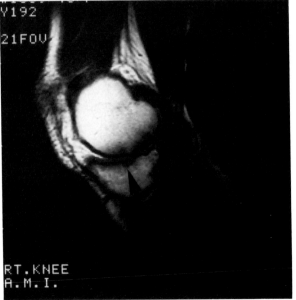

Figure 1 is a coronal view demonstrating the absence of visualization of the meniscus (open arrow). Contrast this to the presence of the lateral meniscus (white arrow). The arrow designates a slight increase in the central portion of the lateral meniscus that represents myxoid degeneration within the meniscal substance. The large arrow demonstrates subchondral changes in the tibial plateau.

In a more posterior coronal cut from the same series, Figure 2 (open arrow) designates the absence of a meniscus medially. The large arrow again demonstrates the changes in the tibial plateau, which include early formation of a subchondral cyst and sclerosis of the bone represented by a decrease in signal along the tibial plateau.

Figure 3, a sagittal cut through the medial meniscus, demonstrates subchondral changes designated by the large arrow. Also note the absence of any visualized meniscus in this image.

2.48 HORIZONTAL MEDIAL MENISCAL TEAR

This 38-year-old male demonstrates severe horizontal tearing of the middle and posterior aspects of the medial meniscus on Figure 1. The large arrow designates increased signal running through the meniscus. Contrast this to the image of the anterior horn (open arrow), which shows a normal dark signal and a triangular shape. Figure 2 demonstrates the horizontal tearing again. There is also some vertical tear that communicates with the inferior surface of the meniscus (arrow). Also, note on Figure 1 the small arrow designating a small area of effusion within the knee.

Figure 3 is a coronal cut through the knee joint contrasting the normal meniscus laterally to the torn, fragmented medial meniscus (open arrow). The laterality can be confirmed on the coronal view by identifying the horizontally oriented posterior cruciate ligament (long-stemmed arrow) with the more vertically oriented anterior cruciate ligament, which is lateral (short arrow).

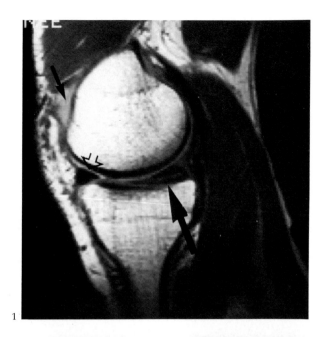

1

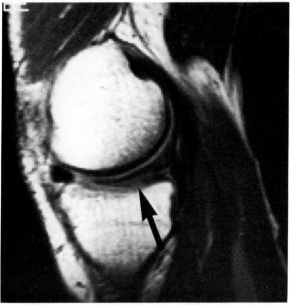

2

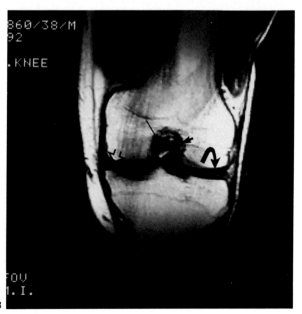

3

2.49 SEVERE MEDIAL COMPARTMENT DEGENERATIVE CHANGES

Figure 1 demonstrates the absence of a medial meniscus (large arrow). Also in this area note the narrowing of the medial compartment, as well as evidence of some osteophytic formation laterally (curved arrow). Sclerotic change in the femora condyle is also evident (long-stemmed arrow). On the coronal image, note the popliteal cyst (open arrow).

Figure 2 represents a slightly more anterior cut through the knee. The curved arrow demonstrates the remnant of the central portion of a medial meniscus. Contrast to this to the more normal preserved lateral meniscus (open arrow).

Figure 3a demonstrates the presence of a small amount of effusion within the joint space (arrow). Open arrows demonstrate the appearance of the popliteal cyst. Figure 3b demonstrates a large amount of material in the joint capsule, posterior and superior to the posterior cruciate ligament (large arrow). This has a heterogeneous signal, and the small arrow points to what may represent a fragment of meniscus within this collection.

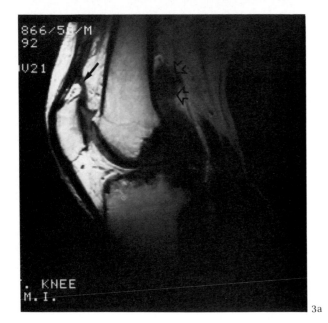

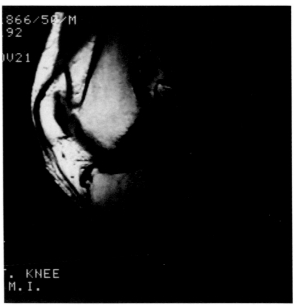

2.50 SMALL POPLITEAL CYST, DESMOID VERSUS SARCOMA

Figure 1 is an axial image demonstrating the intimate relation of this small, fairly well-rounded structure adjacent to the knee. There is even the suggestion of a breech in the knee capsule (curved arrow). Figure 2 demonstrates a sagittal cut through the same structure, again showing its well-circumscribed outer contour and loss of definition in relation to the knee capsule. Figure 3 is a coronal cut demonstrating again the presence of the structure and its intimate relation to the knee capsule.

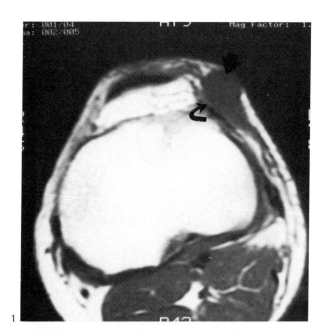

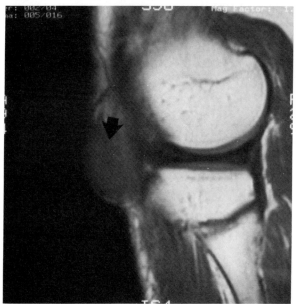

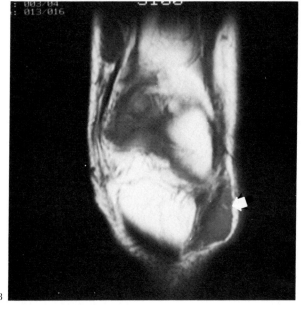

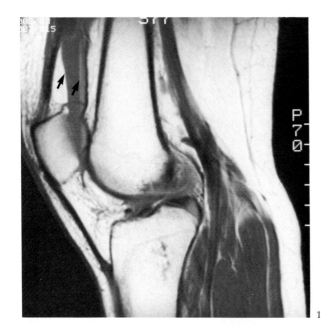

2.51 HEMILIPOARTHROSIS WITH ASSOCIATED LATERAL TIBIAL PLATEAU FRACTURE

Figure 1 demonstrates in the sagittal plane three components of an effusion (small arrows), showing interfaces of the three fluid layers. Fat is floating and is designated by the high signal superiorly. The intermedial fluid represents separation of the hematocrit from the joint fluid. Figures 2 and 3 demonstrate loss of the normal anatomy in the lateral aspect of the lateral plateau (long-stemmed arrows). Also note the diffuse, irregular decrease through the bone marrow representing bone edema.

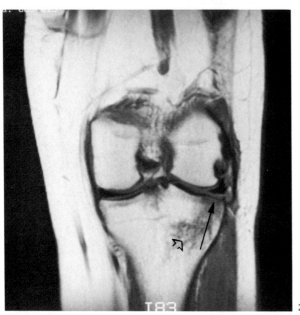

2.52 SMALL POPLITEAL CYST

Figure 1 demonstrates the appearance of a small cyst lateral to the knee joint. Figure 2 again demonstrates this cyst in the axial plane. Note the well-described edge and the suggestion of a small focal area within the knee capsule that may represent the communication between the knee and the cyst, allowing fluid accumulation within the cyst. Figure 3 is a sagittal image (arrow) demonstrating the appearance of the cyst in this plane. Popliteal cysts can occur around any aspect of the knee. These are usually posterior and are referred to as *Baker's cysts*.

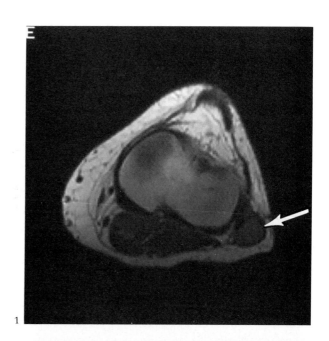

1

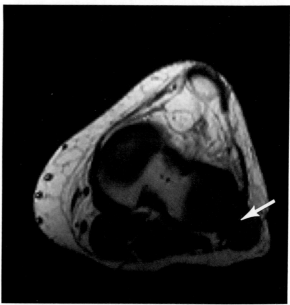

2

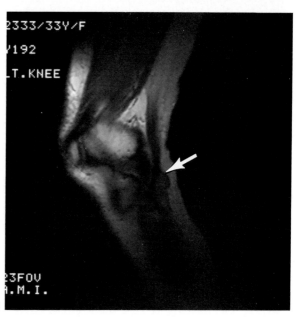

3

2.53 BAKER'S CYST OF THE KNEE

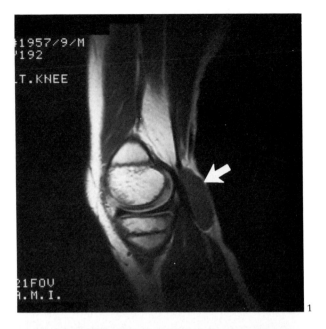

1

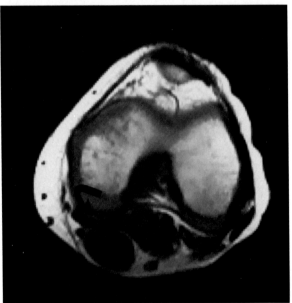

This large Baker's cyst in a 9-year-old male is identified on Figure 1, which represents a sagittal cut through the cyst and knee joint. Figures 2 demonstrates in the axial plane the connection between the cyst and the knee joint, and the defect in the capsule can be identified (curved arrow).

Figure 3 is a coronal image through the cyst demonstrating its relation to the muscle of the upper knee joint (large arrow).

2

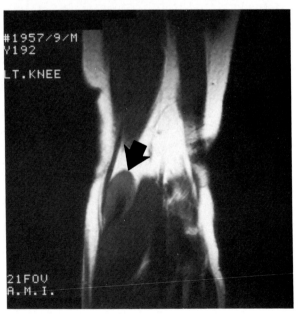

3

2.54 CHONDROMALACIA WITH OSTEOPHYTE INVOLVING THE MEDIAL AND LATERAL COMPARTMENTS

Figure 1 demonstrates the scalloped, irregular appearance of the patellar cartilage. The long arrow demonstrates the scalloped appearance. The short arrow points to the location where the already markedly destroyed and thinned cartilage allows the femoral articular cartilage to touch the subchondral bone.

Figure 2 demonstrates a through-and-through defect of intermediate signal that extends into and beyond the subcortical sclerotic line (long arrow).

Figure 3a demonstrates osteophytes arising from the tibial and femoral surfaces laterally at the knee joints. Figure 3b demonstrates a slightly more anterior cut. The short arrows demonstrate again the appearance of the osteophytes arising from both the medial and lateral condyles. There is also an associated effusion (curved arrow).

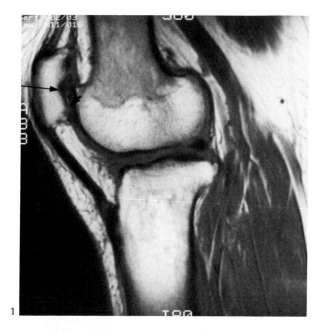

1

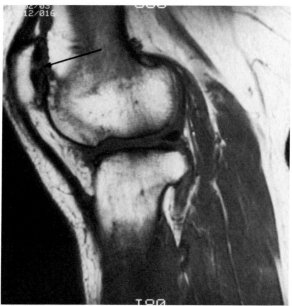

2

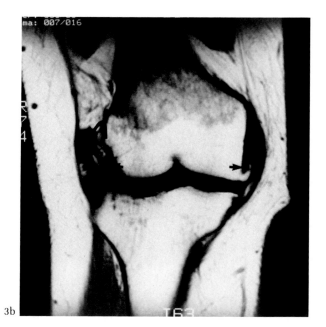

3b

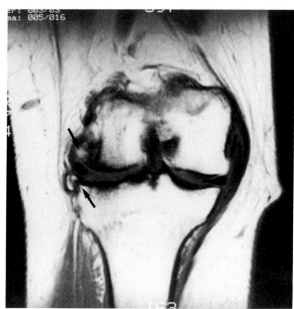

3a

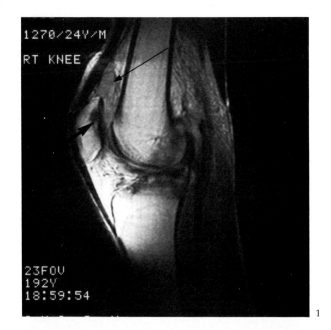

2.55 CHONDROMALACIA WITH EFFUSION

This is a 24-year-old male. An effusion demonstrated on Figures 1 and 2 by a long-stemmed arrow collects in the suprapatellar bursa. The arrows point to the irregular, scalloped appearance of the patella on the sagittal cuts. This scalloped appearance, as well as a subchondral decrease in signal, reflects changes of fairly advanced chondromalacia.

Chondromalacia, or damage to the cartilage, is one of the most common findings in a painful knee in the young adult.

2.56 OSTEOCHONDRITIS DISSECANS

This is a 16-year-old male. Figures 1a and 1b demonstrate alteration of the normal high signal of the epicondyle, showing decreased signal and a suggestion of sclerotic rim (open arrows).

Figure 2 is a coronal cut through this same area of abnormality and demonstrates the same findings. Contrast the altered signal here with that of a normal epiphysis of the femur (arrow).

Figure 3 is an axial representation again demonstrating the osteochondritis defects in the axial plane (open arrows).

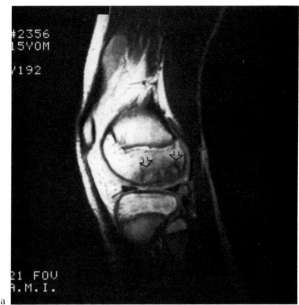

1a

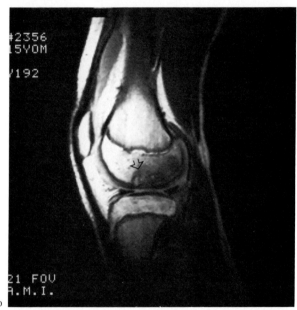

1b

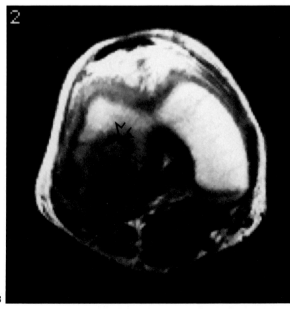

3

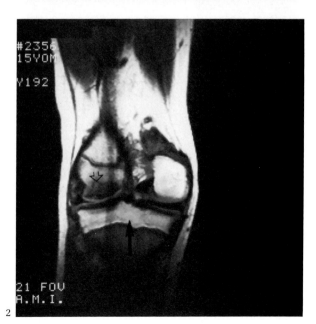

2

2.57 MODERATE CHONDROMALACIA

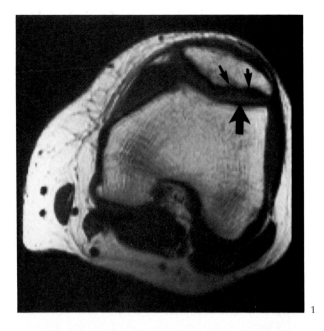

Figure 1 demonstrates thinning of the articular cartilage of the patellar surface (large arrow).

The small arrows demonstrate the scalloped appearance of the bone deep to the cartilage of the patella. Figure 2 again demonstrates that the changes persist on a contiguous axial slice. The patellar articular femoral interface is suggested (long-stemmed arrow). This is lost in the region of the chondromalacia (small arrow).

The sagittal image, Figure 3, demonstrates slight scalloping and irregularity of the subchondral bone (long-stemmed arrows). The small arrow designates a tiny effusion in the suprapatellar bursa.

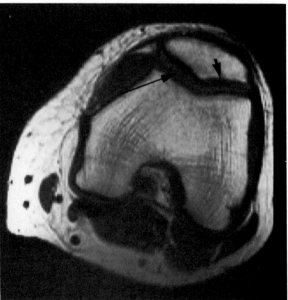

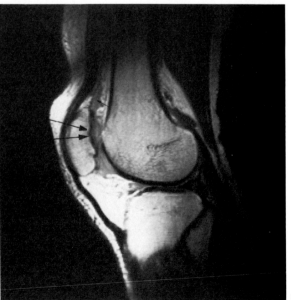

2.58 CHONDROMALACIA OF THE KNEE

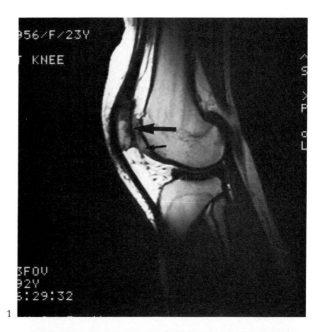

This is a 23-year-old female with a painful knee. Figure 1 demonstrates a subchondral decreased signal within the patella (large arrow). The intact articular cartilage of the femoral condyle can be evaluated (small arrow).

Figure 2 demonstrates the advantage of the axial image over the sagittal image for evaluating the cartilaginous surfaces. The open arrow demonstrates the intact highland cartilage over the femoral condyle. The large white arrow demonstrates the subchondral decreased signal reflecting the subchondral bony reaction to a defect within the overlying cartilaginous surface.

Figure 3 is a cut at a slightly different level through the patella demonstrating the persistence of this focal decrease in signal in the patella immediately deep to the cartilaginous surface.

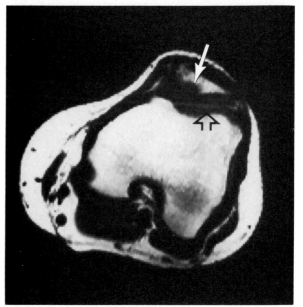

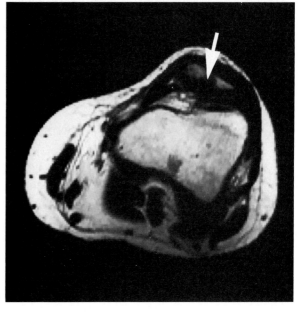

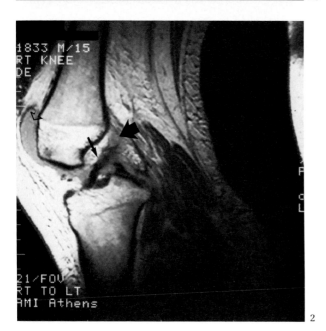
1a

2.59 POSTERIOR AND ANTERIOR CRUCIATE LIGAMENT TEARS

Figure 1a demonstrates the abnormal appearance of the posterior cruciate ligament with numerous tears. The curved arrow designates some of the retained normal signal within the now torn ligament. Figure 1b (curved arrow) again demonstrates, in an additional sagittal cut in the same series, the slightly more distorted appearance of the posterior cruciate ligament. Previous examples have demonstrated the normal appearance of this as a broad, low-signal-intensity structure. The tearing appears to be predominantly midsubstanced and a small arrow on Figure 1b points to the maintenance of at least the tibial attachment of the posterior cruciate ligament.

Figure 2 demonstrates the detachment of the anterior cruciate ligament from the femoral bone (large arrow); the anterior cruciate now has a wavy, slightly formless structure (small arrow). The open arrow demonstrates the presence of an effusion usually associated with cruciate tears.

Figure 3 (curved arrow) demonstrates the distorted, widened appearance of the posterior cruciate ligament, which has now been torn and is interspersed with the hematoma and edema. There are small areas of low signal representing the remaining intact fibers. The open arrow demonstrates the abnormal appearance of the anterior cruciate ligament with similar changes. Note that the relationship between the anterior and posterior cruciate ligaments is still maintained despite tears in both structures.

1b

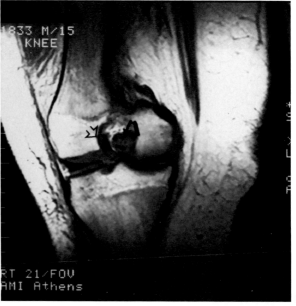

2

3

128

2.60 MARKED CHONDROMALACIA WITH RESULTANT SEVERE OSTEOARTHRITIS

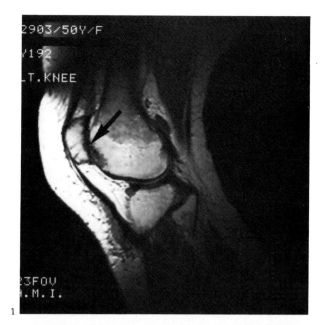

1

The sagittal image, Figure 1, demonstrates marked loss of the normal joint space between the patella and the femoral articular surfaces (large arrow). In addition, note that there is a change in the subchondral bone, represented by loss of signal, reflecting a change within the bony structure.

Figure 2, an axial cut through the patella, demonstrates the narrowing and total destruction of the articular highland cartilage with subchondral sclerosis (small white arrows). The open arrow points to conversion of the normal bone marrow to a higher signal, which suggests a further degenerative reaction of the bone deep to the articular surface. The long-stemmed arrow demonstrates the presence of a small effusion.

Figure 3 is an additional cut demonstrating the lateral subluxation and, more superiorly, an osteophytic-type reaction of the femoral shaft to the degenerative relationship with the patella (short white arrows). The long-stemmed arrow again designates the presence of effusion within the knee joint.

These changes demonstrate the severe destruction that occurred to the cartilaginous surfaces long before any obvious bony reaction could be identified on routine plain films. They also demonstrate that the pathophysiology of osteoarthritis consists primarily of damage to the cartilage, with bone being secondarily damaged by the reaction that is seen. MRI offers new insight into the reactive change occurring in the bone marrow in these areas of arthritis as the bone attempts to react to the changed conditions of the joint.

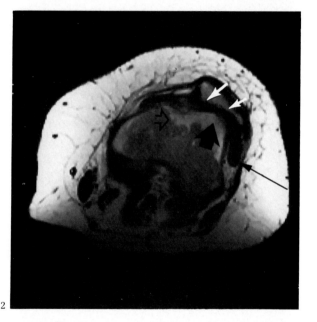

2

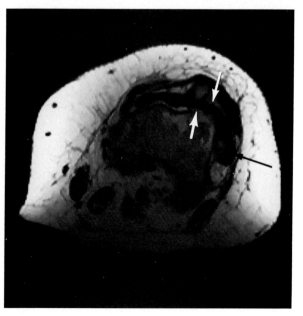

3

2.61 KNEE JOINT MOUSE

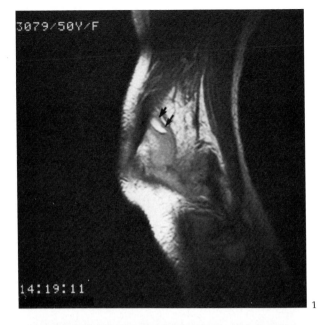

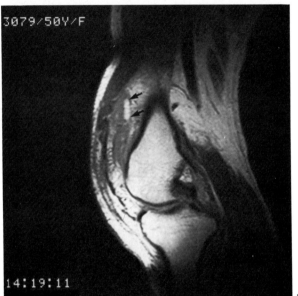

The sagittal images of Figures 1 and 2 demonstrate a high-signal-intensity, well-defined structure floating within the effusion in the suprapatellar bursa (small arrows). This represents a small joint mouse, or fragment of bone within the joint capsule. The axial depiction of this joint mouse is seen on Figures 3a and 3b (large arrow). Note that the joint effusion is easily separated from this high-signal-intensity structure representing free bone. Because of the fat contained within the bone, the bone fragment allows a large amount of contrast between the effusion and the joint mouse. With the absence of any effusion, it is more difficult to identify small joint mice; their signal approaches that of the subcutaneous tissue surrounding the knee joint.

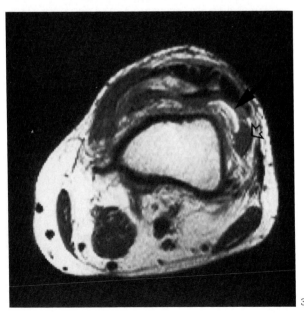

3a

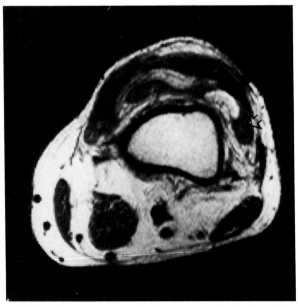

3b

130

2.62 MEDIAL CRUCIATE LIGAMENT TEAR

Figures 1a and 1b demonstrate the coronal appearance of a torn medial collateral ligament. Note the separation of the meniscus from the low-signal, linear structure representing the medial collateral ligament. The curved arrow demonstrates separation of the meniscus from the medial collateral ligament on Figure 1a.

Figures 2 and 3 demonstrate the axial appearance of the tear through the collateral ligament; the lateral aspect of the knee capsule is disrupted. Note that there is a loss of the normal definition of the low-density knee capsule and subcutaneous fat (curved arrows). The open arrow designates joint effusion. Compare the appearance on this axial scan with that of the lateral aspect of the knee (large arrow, Figure 2).

Figure 3, at a slightly different level in the axial plane, again demonstrates disruption of the medial collateral ligament and knee joint (curved arrow).

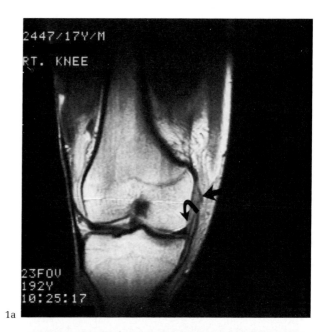
1a

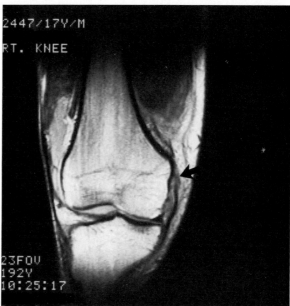
1b

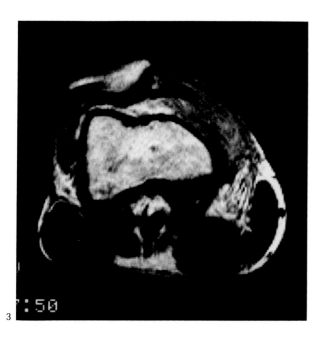
3

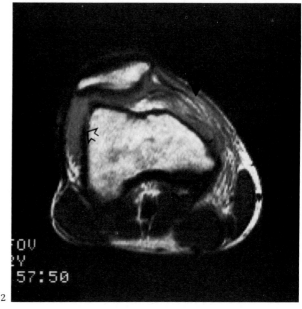
2

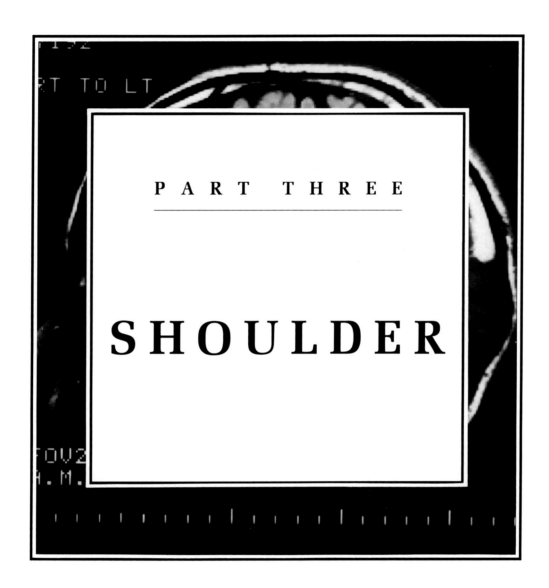

PART THREE

SHOULDER

3.1 ROTATOR CUFF INJURY WITH EFFUSION AND PROBABLE GLENOID LABRUM DAMAGE

Figures 1 to 3 represent coronal images beginning at the most posterior aspect and proceeding anteriorly. On Figure 1 there is evidence in the region of the rotator cuff of discontinuity of the normal low-signal band; this is consistent with a full-thickness tear. This can be seen on all three images and is designated by the large solid arrow. Figures 1 and 2 demonstrate the normal appearance of the superior glenoid labrum (open arrow). The disrupted high signal of the lower lip of the glenoid labrum (curved arrow) suggests tearing of this structure in its inferior portion. The glenoid labrum is similar to the meniscus within the knee. The same criteria used to demonstrate meniscal tears and degeneration apply to the meniscus or glenoid labrum of the shoulder.

These tears and meniscal damage are associated with effusions. On the more T1-weighted image of Figure 3, the effusion is designated as an intermediate "milky" signal adjacent to the humeral head and within the joint space (small solid arrow).

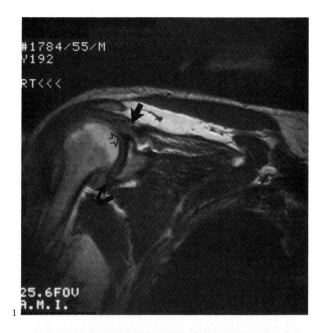

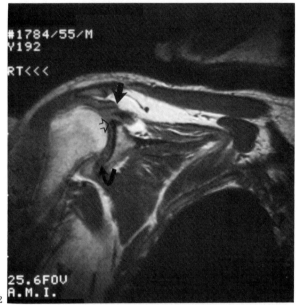

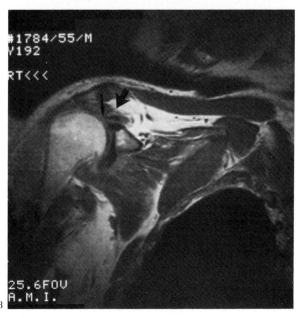

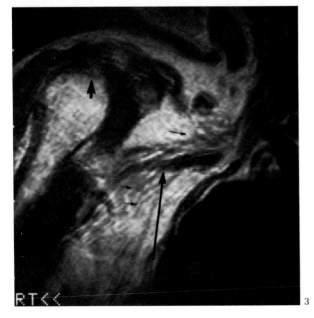

3.2 TORN ROTATOR CUFF STATUS AFTER PRIOR REPAIR

Figure 1 demonstrates the absence of signal void in the region of the superior spinatus tendon that forms a superior aspect of the rotator cuff. This is designated by the long-stemmed arrow. The short arrow points to the partially resected acromioclavicular joint, which has been previously addressed as part of the repair. The normal articular surface is lost, and the acromioclavicular joint is difficult to visualize directly. Figure 2 is another image from this same coronal series, again demonstrating the intermediate signal traversing the superior rotator cuff region. The short arrow demonstrates a slightly more anterior visualization of the more posterior acromioclavicular joint. Figure 3 is an additional coronal image that again demonstrates the defect persisting in the rotator cuff (arrowhead). Additionally, this image demonstrates the subclavian artery, which can be visualized and is designated by the long-stemmed arrow. Close to the subclavian artery is the brachial plexus; the numerous striations of the nerve are suggested in part, running closely around the subclavian (small arrows).

3.3 IMPINGEMENT SYNDROME

Figure 1 demonstrates proliferation of osteophyte along the inferior aspect of the acromioclavicular joint (arrow). Figure 2 is a T2-weighted image documenting the absence of fluid in the subacromial bursa, which suggests that the rotator cuff remains intact. The T2-weighted images are sometimes more useful in adding the increased contrast that allows visualization of the displacement of the rotator cuff and muscle away from the hypertrophic acromioclavicular joint.

Figure 3 demonstrates the chronic defect seen in the superior aspect of the supraspinatus muscle with repeated impingement of the acromioclavicular joint onto the muscle (small arrows).

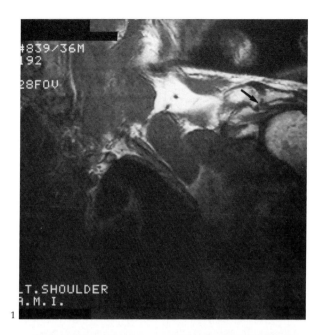

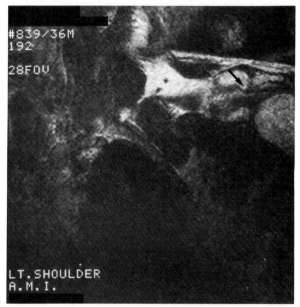

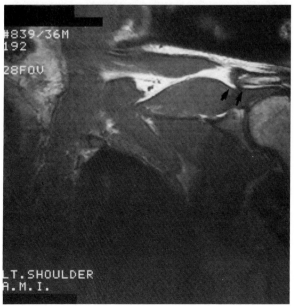

3.4 GLENOID LABRUM TEAR

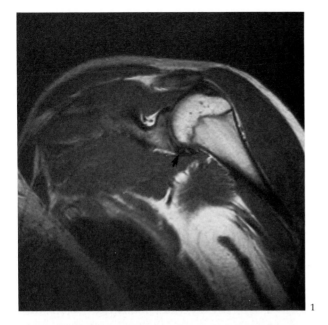

1

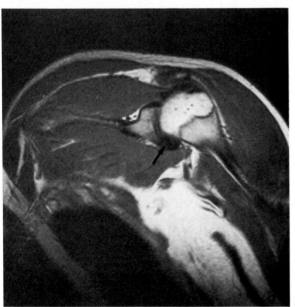

2

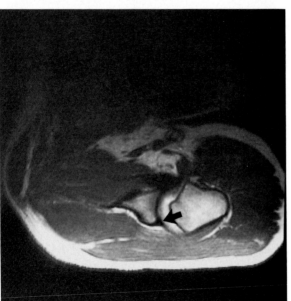

3

Figure 1 demonstrates increased signal within the lower portion of the glenoid labrum (arrow). Figure 2 is a slightly more posterior cut demonstrating additional distortion of the glenoid labrum. The same imaging criteria used for the knee meniscus apply roughly to the glenoid labrum, although the glenoid labrum is more difficult to visualize as directly as the knee. We like to employ at least three views of the shoulder in the coronal, axial, and sagittal planes for visualization and inspection of all the structures of the shoulder. Figure 3 demonstrates the distortion of the anterior portion of the glenoid labrum in the region shown on the sagittal views. Compare this to the more posterior aspect of the glenoid, which is maintaining a normal triangular low signal (solid arrow).

3.5 IMPINGEMENT SYNDROME SECONDARY TO TRAUMA

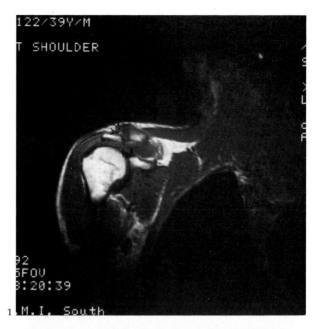

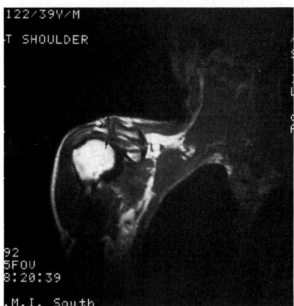

This is a 39-year-old male with a previous acromioclavicular dislocation. Figure 1 demonstrates the slight disruption of the acromioclavicular joint (open arrow). This disruption and the reactive fluid surrounding its healing have produced a mass effect on the supraspinatus muscle. Small arrows indicate the intact rotator cuff. Figure 2 again demonstrates, in a slightly more anterior cut, the prominence of the acromioclavicular joint following this trauma. The small arrow indicates a small area of intermediate signal that traverses the rotator cuff. Some concern was raised about the presence of a small partial tear within the cuff at this level.

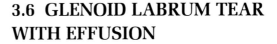

3.6 GLENOID LABRUM TEAR WITH EFFUSION

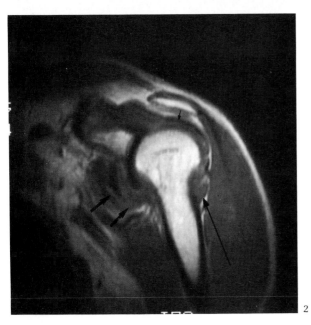

This is a 42-year-old male. An effusion is present on Figure 1a and is represented by an open arrow. The glenoid labrum has been torn and is displaced in a medial posterior fashion (long-stemmed arrow). Note the visualization of the biceps tendon (small arrow). Figure 1b demonstrates, in a more inferior cut, continued damage of the glenoid labrum and visualization of a tear through this portion of the labrum, which has not been displaced. The open arrow again identifies effusion within the joint. Figure 2 demonstrates displacement of the axillary recess (arrows). The long-stemmed arrow demonstrates effusion along the lateral aspect of the humeral shaft proximally. The small arrow demonstrates visualization of the rotator cuff, which appears intact.

Figure 3 demonstrates an increased signal of the effusion (small arrows) on a T2-weighted image.

1a

1b

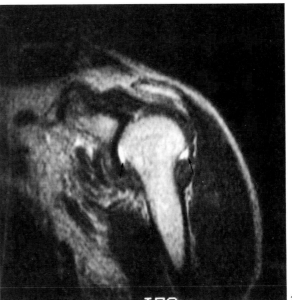

2

3

3.7 ROTATOR CUFF INJURY FOLLOWING TRAUMA

This 53-year-old male fell and developed acute pain in the shoulder. Figure 1 demonstrates disruption of the rotator cuff (large arrow). Maintenance of the tendon's insertion into the muscle is suggested by the small arrow. The arrows with stems point to the glenoid labrum, which appears normal except for a tiny amount of signal in the inferior portion, which may represent some intrameniscal degenerative change. Figure 2 again confirms the disrupted, torn appearance of the rotator cuff (large arrow); the long-stemmed arrow also demonstrates the good visualization of the meniscus.

Figure 3a is a T2-weighted image again demonstrating the appearance of the torn rotator cuff. Figure 3b is a sagittal cut through the same shoulder, demonstrating absence of an identifiable low-signal structure representing the rotator cuff at this level. This region contains an intermediate signal that is consistent with diffuse posttraumatic fluid, and possibly some hemorrhage.

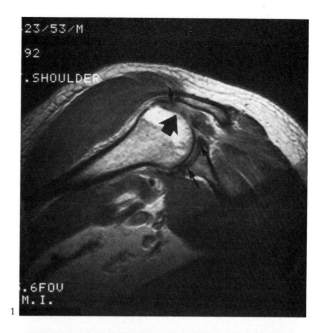

1

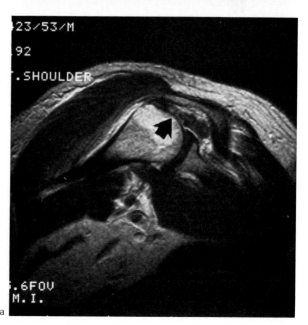

2

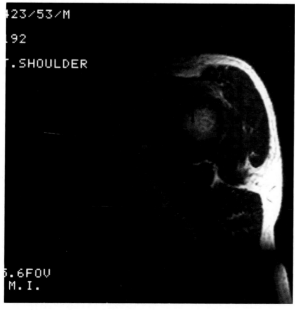

3b

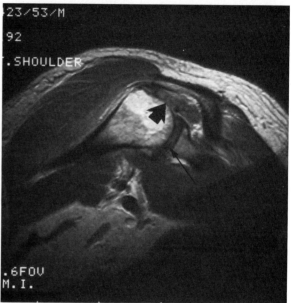

3a

3.8 LIPOMA OF THE UPPER EXTREMITY

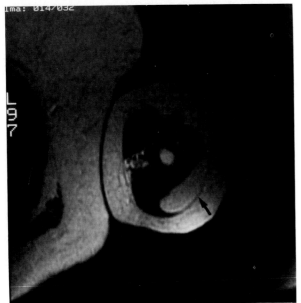

This is an intramuscular lipoma. Figure 1 is a coronal cut through the upper extremity demonstrating the fatty tumor residing within the muscle of the triceps (arrows). Figure 2 is an axial cut demonstrating good delineation of the intramuscular lipoma, as well as a fibrous capsule or possibly some residual muscle fiber extending over the lipoma and separating it from the abundant subcutaneous tissues within the upper arm. Figure 3, a T2-weighted image, demonstrates signal suppression of the fat in both the lipoma and the subcutaneous tissue, allowing the confident diagnosis that this tumor is composed primarily of fat.

3.9 OSTEOARTHRITIS
OF THE SHOULDER

Figure 1 demonstrates marked loss of the normal humeral glenoid labrum articulation (arrows). The signal change represents fairly marked osteoarthritis.

   Figure 2 demonstrates the torn, distorted glenoid labrum (arrow). Figure 3 demonstrates effusion within the joint. As with the abnormality seen in the knee, as the meniscus is destroyed, the underlying bone interacts and reacts in an osteoarthritic manner. The destructive changes are fairly marked in this example. Only fragments of the glenoid labrum can still be identified (Figure 2, arrow).

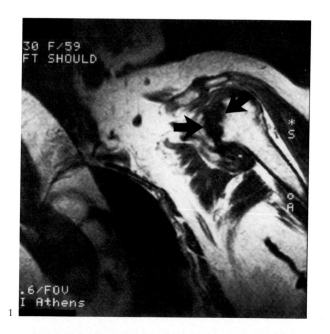

1

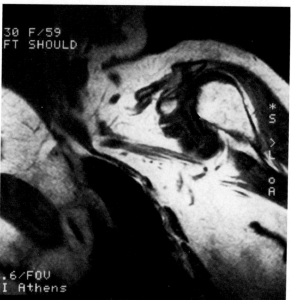

2

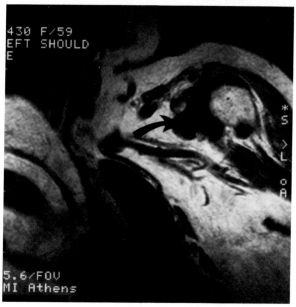

3

3.10 ACROMIOCLAVICULAR TRAUMATIC SEPARATION

This is a 36-year-old male with a recent shoulder injury and acromioclavicular separation clinically. Figures 1a and 1b are coronal images demonstrating separation of the acromioclavicular joint, with fluid surrounding the joint space (large arrows). The shoulder joint also has an effusion, and the axillary recess is distended (long-stemmed white arrow).

Figures 2a and 2b are T2-weighted images enhancing the fluid in the traumatically separated acromioclavicular joint. Figure 3 demonstrates the blunted, distorted appearance of the meniscus of the glenoid labrum, which is consistent with a tear at this level. The curved arrow points to the intact normal posterior horn of the glenoid labrum.

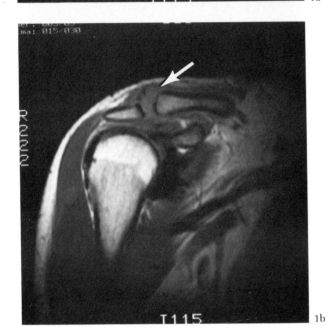

1a

1b

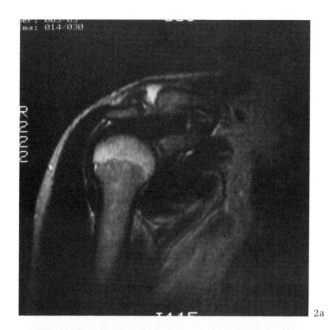

2a

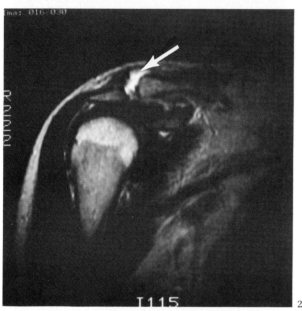

2b

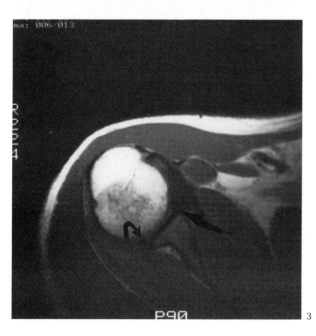

3

145

3.11 IMPINGEMENT SYNDROME WITH ROTATOR CUFF TEAR

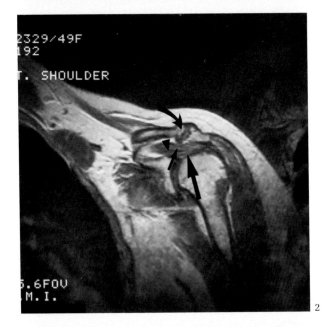

This is a 49-year-old female with an impingement syndrome. Figure 1 demonstrates osteophytic change within the acromioclavicular joint (arrow).

Figure 2 (curved arrow) demonstrates the osteophyte. Note its impingement on the supraspinatus muscle (small arrow).

The rotator cuff is incomplete, as demonstrated by the intermediate signal through a normally low-signal structure (large arrow). Some of the retracted rotator cuff can be seen (arrowhead).

The interrupted rotator cuff is again designated by an arrowhead, and the interruption is pointed to by a large arrow in Figure 3, which is a slightly more anterior cut. Effusion in the axillary recess is indicated by the curved arrow.

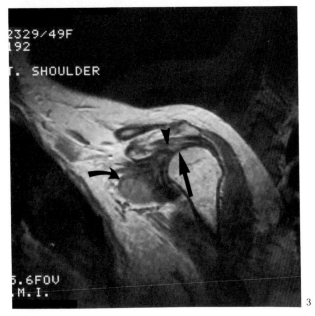

3.12 FRACTURED HUMERAL HEAD WITH SHOULDER EFFUSION AND DAMAGE TO THE GLENOID LABRUM

This is an 82-year-old female with a fractured humerus demonstrated on the coronal image (Figure 1, curved arrow). There is an associated effusion (open arrows) that distends the superior portion of the rotator cuff upward (arrowhead).

Figure 2 is a T2-weighted image enhancing the effusion. The changes identified on Figure 1 are seen. The effusions, represented by open arrows, demonstrate that the rotator cuff is displaced superiorly (arrow). The fracture line is not as well as seen with the T2 image (curved arrow). Figure 3 demonstrates increased signal in the anterior portion of the glenoid labrum, reflecting damage within the meniscus. The open arrow again demonstrates the appearance of the effusion separating the humeral head from the glenoid (open arrow).

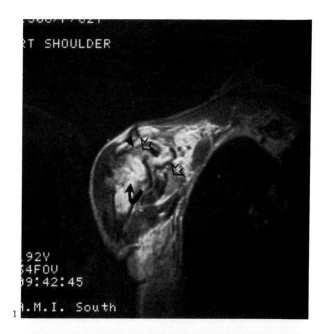

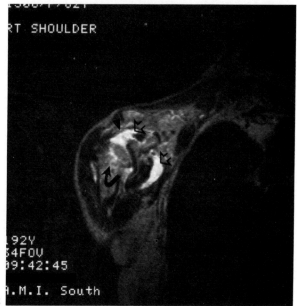

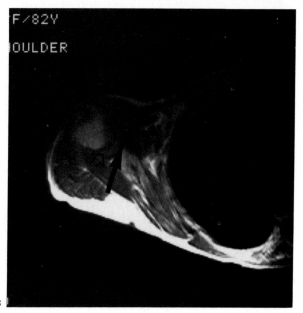

147

3.13 TORN GLENOID LABRUM

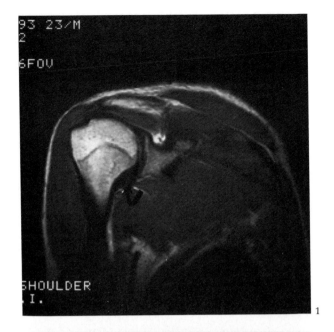

1

This is a 23-year-old male with a painful shoulder following a recent injury. Figure 1 demonstrates complex tearing through the inferior lip of the glenoid labrum (curved arrow). Figure 2 is a sagittal cut through the lower lip of the glenoid. As with the knee meniscus, this should be a homogeneous low signal. Alteration of the signal suggests damage within the disc or tearing that communicates with the articular surface through the disc material. Figures 3a and 3b demonstrate the tears in the axial plane through the lower glenoid labrum (arrows).

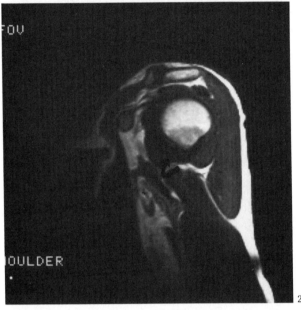

2

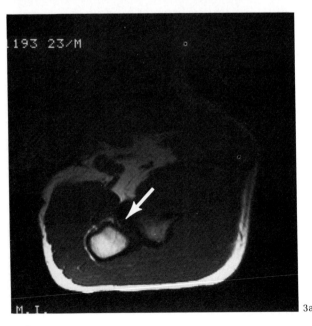

3a

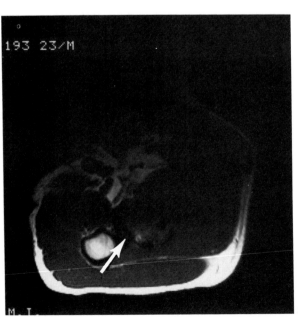

3b

3.14 SHOULDER IMPINGEMENT SYNDROME

This is a 47-year-old female with clinical presentation of shoulder impingement. Figure 1a demonstrates a large osteophyte that extends into the superior rotator cuff. Figure 2 is a zoom-up, or magnified view, demonstrating the alteration of the rotator cuff (arrowheads) and the relationship of the cuff and muscle to the large osteophyte (arrow). Note incidentally the nicely demonstrated glenoid labrum (curved arrow). Figure 1b demonstrates a slight defect in the superior portion of the suprascapularis muscle following chronic impingement by the osteophyte.

Figure 3 (curved arrow) demonstrates the hypertrophic change in the acromioclavicular joint in the sagittal plane (arrowheads demonstrate the thinning of the cuff and muscle at this level).

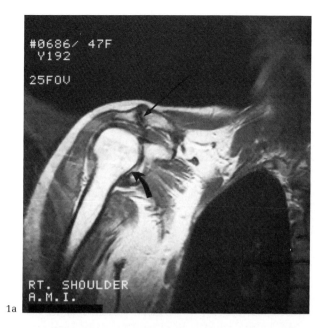

1a

1b

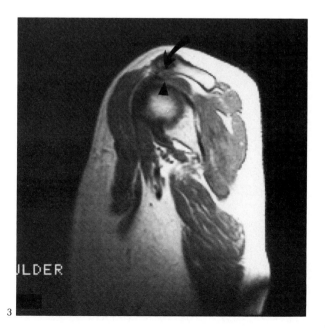

3

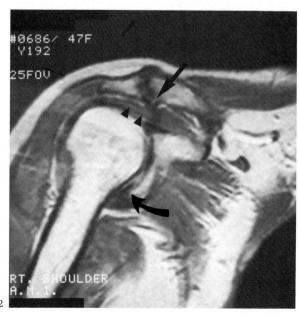

2

3.15 ROTATOR CUFF TEAR WITH SMALL SUBACROMIAL EFFUSION

Figure 1 is a T1-weighted image in the coronal plane through the shoulder joint demonstrating a defect in the normally low-signal rotator cuff. Figure 2 is a T2-weighted image at the same level confirming the presence of loss of normal signal void with intermediate signal traversing the rotator cuff. Figure 3a is a proton density-weighted image demonstrating a small, circular collection in the subacromial bursa. Figure 3b shows increased signal in this region, where the remaining subcutaneous fat shows decreased signal; this appearance suggests a small effusion. The presence of a small subacromial effusion and the demonstration of direct visualization of interruption of the rotator cuff allow a confident diagnosis of a rotator cuff injury.

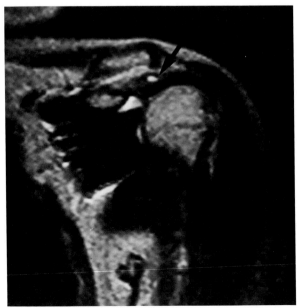

1

2

3a

3b

3.16 IMPINGEMENT SYNDROME WITH SUGGESTION OF CHRONIC DAMAGE TO THE ROTATOR CUFF

Figure 1 (curved arrow) demonstrates a large osteophyte in the acromioclavicular joint. There is poor definition of the rotator cuff (open arrow). Figure 2 is a T2-weighted image through the same level, again demonstrating the osteophyte and absence of visualization of a normal rotator cuff structure. This image shows no evidence of fluid in the subacromial bursa, which makes definitive diagnosis of a tear more difficult.

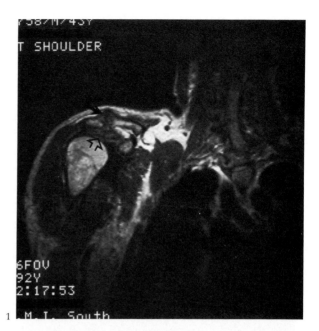

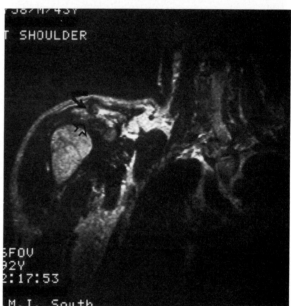

3.17 IMPACTION FRACTURE WITH IMPINGEMENT SYNDROME AND JOINT EFFUSION

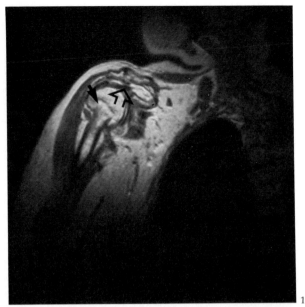

1

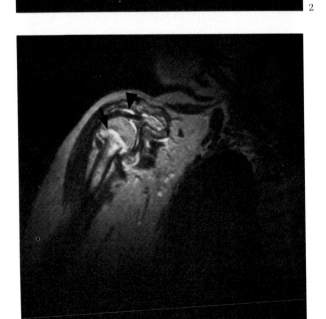

2

Figure 1 demonstrates a large osteophyte arising from the inferior acromioclavicular joint indenting the rotator cuff (open arrow). Note the presence of an impaction fracture of the shaft in the humeral head (small solid arrow).

Figure 2 again demonstrates the mass effect of the osteophyte into the rotator cuff. The open arrow demonstrates the visualization on the T2-weighted image of the glenoid labrum.

Figure 3 again demonstrates the impaction fracture and shows fluid superior to the rotator cuff (arrowhead). Fluid in the subacromial bursa is a secondary sign indicating damage to the rotator cuff. In the presence of a fracture, this finding is less specific.

Figure 4 (curved arrow) demonstrates the presence of fusion within the axillary recess. The small arrow again demonstrates the cortical disruption of the shaft and humeral head secondary to the impaction fracture.

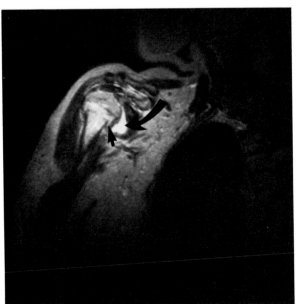

3

4

152

3.18 IMPINGEMENT SYNDROME RIGHT SHOULDER

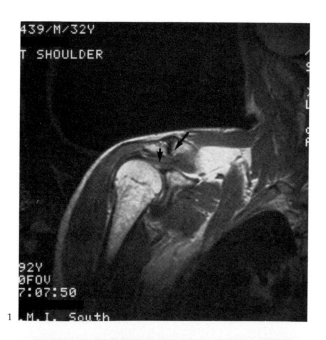

This is a 32-year-old male with a painful right shoulder that cannot be moved. Figure 1 demonstrates a hypertrophic acromioclavicular joint (small arrow). The arrowhead shows the presence of low signal in the midsuperior rotator cuff. Figure 2, a more anterior coronal cut from this same sequence, demonstrates slight irregularity of the more lateral rotator cuff; this suggests a partial tear through the rotator cuff. It is implied that the hypertrophic changes of the acromioclavicular joint cause repetitive trauma to the superior rotator cuff that results in tearing. Figure 3a is a T2-weighted image that demonstrates high signal superior to the supraspinatous muscle and within the subacromial bursa representing effusion. This is a secondary sign of rotator cuff injury. Figure 3b again demonstrates the defect caused by the osteophyte at the acromioclavicular joint. The small arrow indicates the supraspinatus muscle as it is being indented by the hypertrophic acromioclavicular joint.

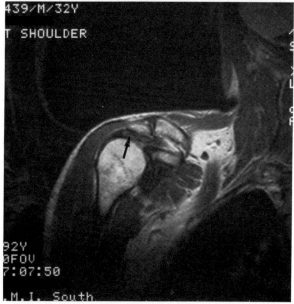

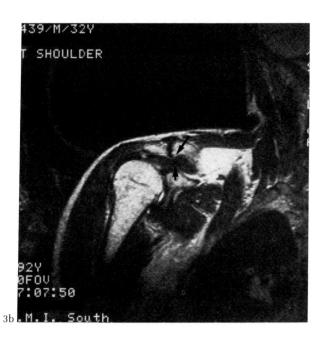

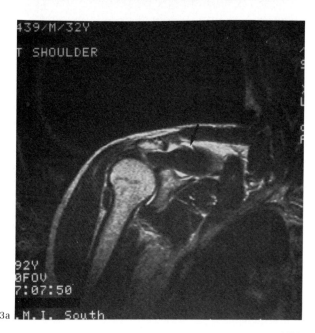

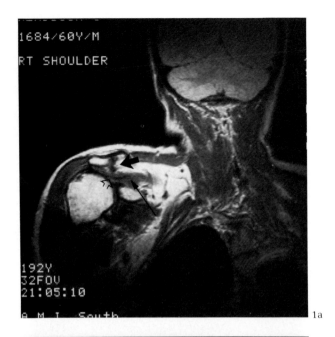

1a

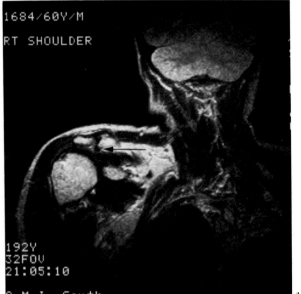

1b

3.19 IMPINGEMENT SYNDROME SECONDARY TO OSTEOPHYTE OF THE RIGHT SHOULDER

This is a 60-year-old male. Figures 1a and 1b demonstrate a large osteophyte extending off the inferior surface of the acromioclavicular joint (large arrow). The open arrow demonstrates the rotator cuff, which is deviated downward secondary to the presence of the osteophyte. The belly of the supraspinatus muscle, designated by the large, long-stemmed arrow, demonstrates the mass effect of the osteophyte and the slight retraction of the muscle fibers. Chronic, progressive damage can result in a signal change in the portion of the muscle adjacent to the osteophyte reflecting both scar and fatty atrophy. Figure 1b is a T2-weighted image that shows, to slightly better effect, the presence of the osteophyte within the fat in relation to the superior portion of the supraspinatus muscle and the rotator cuff (long-stemmed arrow).

Figure 2 is another T1-weighted image from the coronal series, again demonstrating the downward effect of the osteophyte (large arrow) on the rotator cuff (open arrow). Figure 3 is a sagittal representation. The arrow demonstrates the hypertrophic change in the acromioclavicular joint, and the curved arrow points to the interface between the muscle and the osteophyte as the osteophyte impinges on the muscle bundle at this level, as well as on a portion of the muscle bundle at this level of the sagittal cut through the same shoulder.

The rotator cuff can be demonstrated as intact. MRI is also exquisitely sensitive in demonstrating and detecting the status of the muscle, particularly the supraspinatus muscle, at this level. The impingement syndrome is well known to the orthopedic surgeon; however, direct visualization and documentation of the status of the acromioclavicular joint and rotator cuff is one of the newer areas of MRI imaging. Arthrography can demonstrate tears of the cuff, but the actual impingement and direct visualization of these relationships cannot be demonstrated as dramatically.

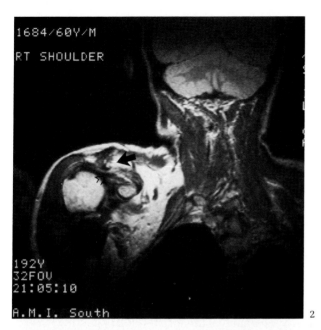

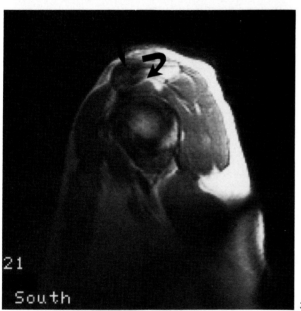

3.20 ROTATOR CUFF TEAR

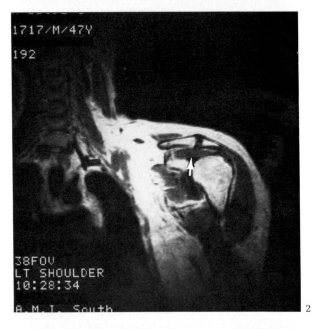

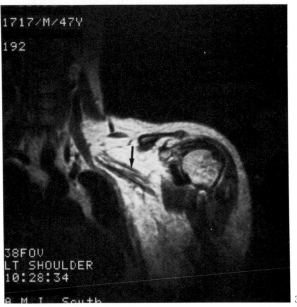

Figure 1 demonstrates the incomplete appearance of the rotator cuff (large arrow). Note the slightly retractile and redundant quality of the muscle and the more proximal tendinous fibers (short arrow). The direct visualization of a break within the normally low-signal structure is the best identification of a rotator cuff injury. Partial tears are more difficult to ascertain. Inspection of the T2 images, particularly for the secondary sign of fluid in the subacromial bursa, is useful.

Figure 2 demonstrates again some of the redundant, heterogeneous appearance of the torn tendon retracting toward the supraspinatous muscle (arrow).

In Figure 1, the tiny arrows demonstrate visualization of the subclavian artery, and the large, long-stemmed arrow demonstrates the brachial plexus nerves as they wrap closely around the subclavian artery. Figure 3 again demonstrates, in a slightly more anterior cut, the relationship of the subclavian artery to the brachial plexus (arrow).

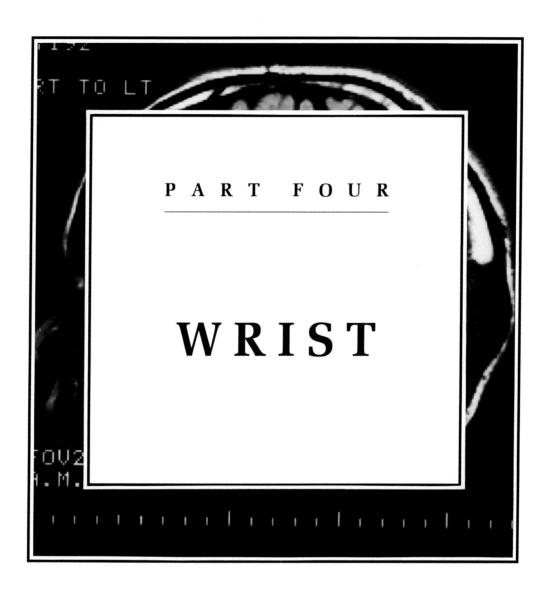

PART FOUR

WRIST

4.1 TENDON SHEATH CYST VERSUS HEMATOMA

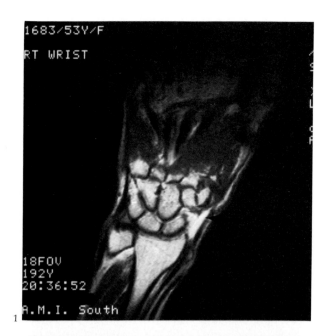

1683/53Y/F
RT WRIST
18FOV
192Y
20:36:52
A.M.I. South

This is a 53-year-old female with focal pain that correlates with the area along the medial aspect of the left wrist (Figure 1, arrow). There is a curvilinear, fairly well-defined area of increased signal that follows along the tendon in this area and is consistent with a tendon sheath cyst or possibly a hematoma.

Figures 2 and 3 (large arrows) point to the cyst that appears to be adjacent to the extensor pollicis brevis. Figure 4 demonstrates the ulnar shaft, designated by the long-stemmed arrow. The T2-weighted image shows slight enhancement in the area of abnormality.

1

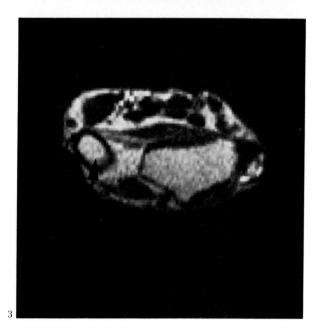

2

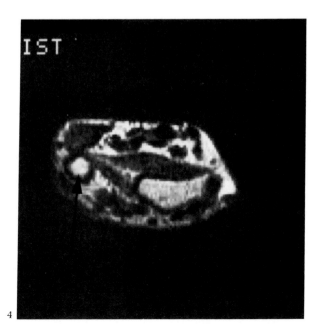

4

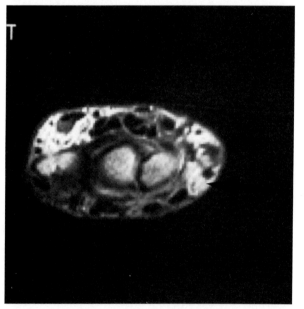

3

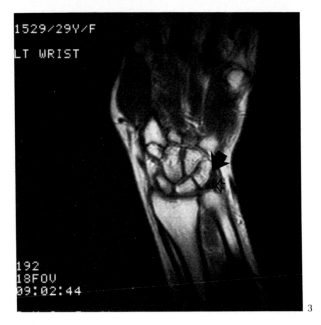

4.2 CARPAL TUNNEL SYNDROME

This is a 29-year-old female with clinical findings of carpal tunnel syndrome. Figure 1 demonstrates the tight appearance of the tendons as they pass through the carpal tunnel (large arrow).

Figure 2 is a zoom-up view of the axial views. The long-stemmed arrow points to the hook of the hamate, which delineates the most pertinent level at which to observe the carpal tunnel. The large short-stemmed arrow points to the area of the median nerve, which is prominent; this suggests mild swelling, which is an important part of the diagnosis by MRI criteria of the carpal tunnel syndrome. I have found that inspection of the carpal tunnel region and the close positioning of the tendons are easily documented. Despite the literature on the median nerve, edema is not as apparent in cases I have encountered as I would have hoped; some of our patients have had a profound clinical median nerve presentation without significant enlargement of the nerve. This may be related to the timeliness of the image and the onset of the symptoms.

Figure 3 demonstrates (open arrow) the triangular cartilage. In this patient, it was documented as a routine part of the wrist exam. The triangular cartilage can undergo trauma much like that at the knee meniscus. The same rule of visualizing low-density triangular cartilage and inspecting for increased signal, which may represent tear, can be applied to this cartilaginous structure, as well as to the knee.

4.3 WRIST STATUS AFTER CARPAL TUNNEL RELEASE

Figure 1 is an axial cut at the level of the hook of the hamate (curved arrow). The large arrow points to the released retinaculum. Note that the tendons dip slightly toward the palmar surface (large arrow).

Figure 2 is a coronal cut through the wrist. Note that the hamate can be visualized (arrow). Also note that there is a small amount of signal between the tendons, suggesting that they are no longer crowded by a tight retinaculum. Figure 3 demonstrates the absence of any increased signal or swelling of the median nerve, suggesting that the release has been successful.

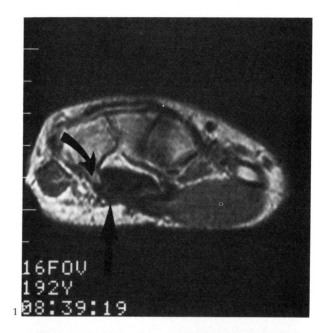

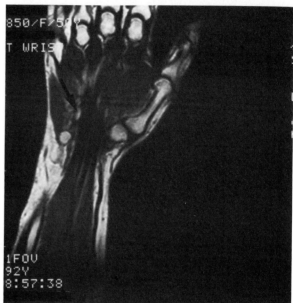

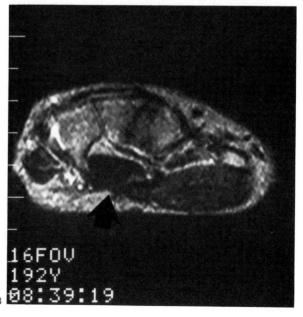

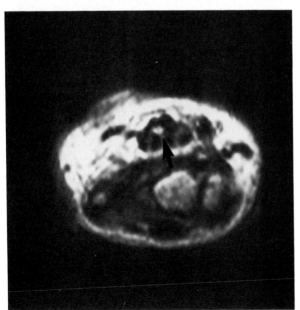

4.4 POSSIBLE CARPAL TUNNEL SYNDROME

This is a less definitive case. Figure 1 demonstrates a slight bunching in the coronal plane of the tendons at the level of the carpal tunnel (arrows). However, the axial images in Figures 1 and 2 demonstrate a more loose grouping of the tendons than is seen on some of the carpal tunnel examples presented. There is more fascial and fatty tissue between the tendons. Figures 3 and 4 (arrow) may be pointing to the slightly enlarged nerve, but a definitely edematous median nerve cannot be demonstrated. Figure 2 (arrow) demonstrates the level of the hook of the hamate, which is a good bony landmark for the region of the carpal tunnel.

Carpal tunnel release involves releasing the flexor retinaculum, allowing more movement of the tendons and taking pressure off the median nerve to relieve the median palsy. However, if visualization suggests that the tendons at the level of the carpal tunnel are somewhat loose and there is adequate space, the diagnosis of carpal tunnel syndrome becomes somewhat more suspect. Up to now, only plain film radiographs, including a shoot-through view of the carpal tunnel, were available to assess the overall dimensions of the carpal tunnel. We now have the ability to image the carpal tunnel in several planes, and, more importantly, to visually inspect the tendons and their association with each other, as well as the median nerve, for evaluation of edema, which is conclusive proof of nerve irritation.

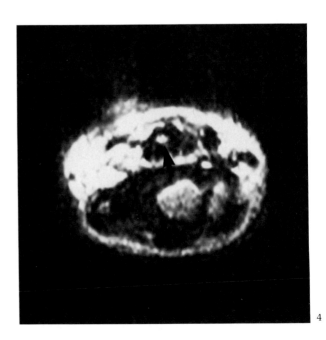

4.5 FRACTURE AND AVASCULAR NECROSIS OF THE NAVICULAR BONE

This is a patient who sustained trauma to the wrist. Characteristic signal loss consistent with avascular necrosis is evident in the navicular bone (large arrow). Comparison of the lunate with a normal signal is seen in Figure 1 (small arrow). The presence of avascular necrosis and a fractured navicular bone is related to the location of the fracture and to the blood supply of the navicular bone. The appearance of an avascular necrosis in the navicular bone is a useful clinical finding for appropriate management.

Figure 2 is an additional coronal cut through the navicular bone. The curved arrow delineates a fracture through the waist and head of the bone. The large arrow again demonstrates a diffuse low signal of the navicular bone, which is consistent with avascular necrosis. This can be contrasted to the adjacent lunate bone (small arrow).

Figure 3 is a less useful motion-degraded axial image that shows the appearance of the decreased signal in the avascular necrosis-affected navicular bone (large arrow).

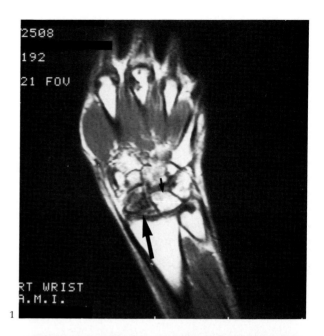

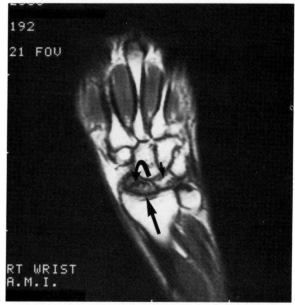

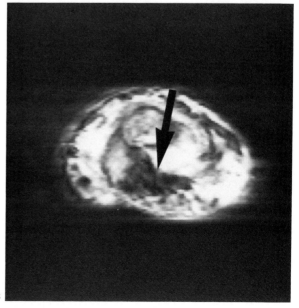

163

4.6 LARGE HEMANGIOMA OF THE WRIST

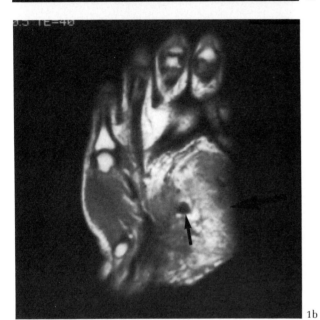

1a

1b

This is a 40-year-old female with a mass in the wrist. Figures 1a and 1b are coronal cuts through a very large soft tissue mass that infiltrates between the muscle and tendinous fibers (arrows). The small arrow demonstrates a low signal centrally that may represent some focal hemorrhage or a tiny metal foreign body, possibly a small clip from a previous surgical procedure. Figures 2a and 2b are sagittal cuts through this mass, which has poorly defined edges and a large amount of interstitial stroma. The appearance is most suggestive of a sarcoma of the muscle, possibly arising from the thenar muscles. Such large, bulky tumors with diffuse interstitial structure could also represent a capillary form of hemangioma. A history of longevity in a tumor of this size, as well as any pertinent changes, such as pain or a change in the size of the tumor, would also be useful in clinical staging of such tumors.

Figure 3 is a T2-enhanced coronal cut demonstrating the extent of the tumor as it interdigitates between the tendons of the extensor muscles of the palm and showing a very bright increase in signal.

The differential diagnosis is between a sarcoma and a very large hemangioma, possibly with sarcomatous elements. The case illustrates the diffuse involvement of the tumor and its extensive interdigitation with major ligamentous structures of the wrist. Note that despite the tumor's fairly involved appearance, there is no underlying bone abnormality. On the basis of T1- and T2-weighted characteristics alone, it would be difficult to differentiate further between a sarcoma and a hemangioma.

This case is through the courtesy of Dr. Robert Chiteman of Maryland Magnetic Imaging.

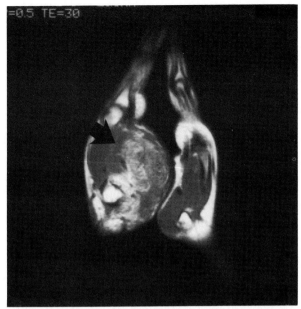

2a

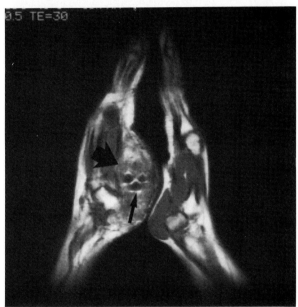

2b

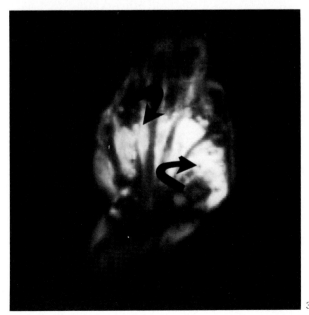

3

165

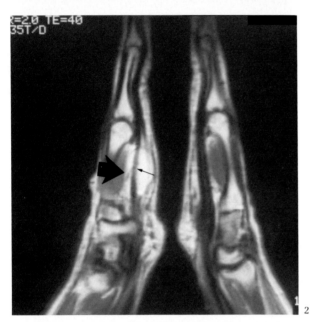

4.7 FLEXOR TENDON GANGLION CYST

Figure 1 demonstrates a well-circumscribed, high-signal cyst surrounding the tendon (small arrow). The large arrow points to the outer lateral limits of the tendinous cyst. Figure 2 is a sagittal cut again demonstrating the tendon surrounded by the cyst (large arrow). The tendon is nicely outlined in this cut (small arrow).

Figure 3 is an axial cut demonstrating again the relationship of the cyst as it surrounds the tendon. These small tendon cysts can be nicely visualized with MRI, and given the numerous plains of imaging, the relationship to the tendon is unparalleled. Most importantly, the cyst is homogeneous, with a well-defined border, allowing exclusion of any underlying soft tissue elements that would raise the possibility of a sarcoma rather than a simple cyst.

This case is through the courtesy of Dr. Robert Chiteman of Maryland Magnetic Imaging.

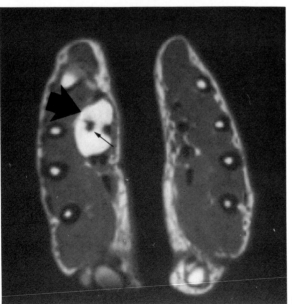

4.8 DEGENERATIVE OSTEOARTHRITIS OF THE NAVICULAR LUNATE JOINT

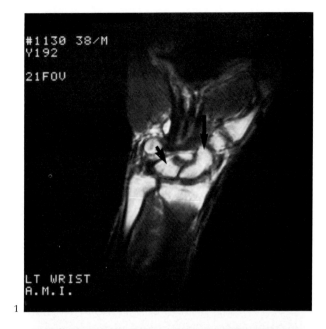

This is a 38-year-old male with a painful wrist. Figure 1 (long arrow) points to the navicular bone. The short arrow points to the lunate joint. This is a coronal view through the wrist. Figure 2 demonstrates the slightly different level of the articulation between the carpal bones. There is a slight loss of the normally sharp delineation seen on Figure 1.

Figures 3 and 4 demonstrate the loss of the joint space, as well as some osteophytic lipping (long-stemmed arrows). This is consistent with an osteoarthritic change within this joint.

The use of MRI for the diagnosis of osteoarthritis in its current state is probably excessive. However, plain films show the end result of osteoarthritis, the reaction of bone following damage of the outer cartilaginous surface. In this case, the other procedure that could be used to show such changes is an axial CT scan, which may underestimate some of the soft tissue changes that may be present. The usual workup following the history, physical exam, and plain films is still equivocal or misunderstood but is suggestive of joint abnormality. MRI focused on the area of concern can sometimes yield useful results, such as those shown here.

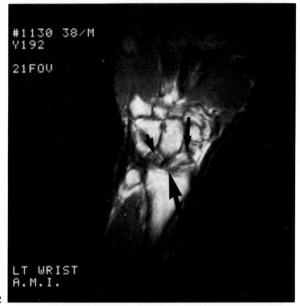

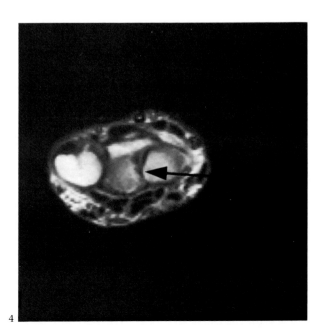

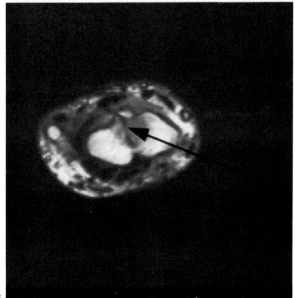

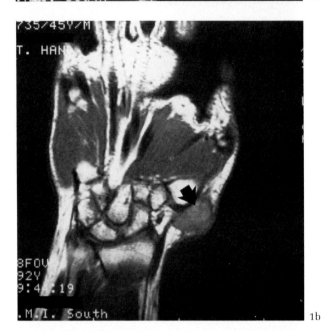

1a

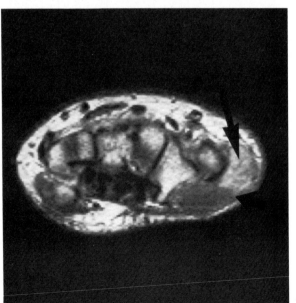

1b

4.9 THENAR MUSCLE MASS, POSSIBLE SARCOMA

Figures 1a and 1b demonstrate, in the coronal plane, a soft tissue-type mass arising immediately lateral to the tendon adjacent to the thenar muscle. The curved arrow on Figure 1a demonstrates the superior extent of the tumor. The large arrow demonstrates a displaced tendon immediately medial to the mass. On Figure 2, the arrow is pointing to the actual mass, which is an intermediate signal only slightly higher than that of the normal muscle in the surrounding wrist region.

Figure 2 is an axial cut through the mass. The large arrow points to the mass. The short-stemmed arrow points to the interface between the mass and the muscle. The muscle appears to be resting against the mass, and the poor interface suggests that the tumor may be arising from the muscle, as seen with sarcoma. Figure 3 is an axial cut through the largest portion of the mass, demonstrating the involvement of the other structures except the single tendon adjacent to the mass.

Figure 4 is a T2-weighted image that shows no significant increase in signal in the mass.

The differential diagnosis would be a low-grade sarcoma. This is not consistent with a tendon cyst or a hematoma. The loss of interface between the thenar muscle and this mass is the strongest evidence suggesting low-grade sarcoma in this region. A neuroma should exhibit a pronounced increase in signal on a T2-weighted image, since this is not present the diagnosis of a neuroma is much less likely (see Figure 4).

2

168

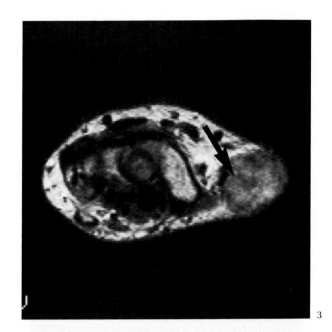

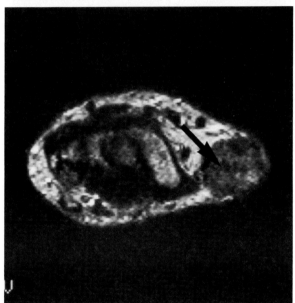

4.10 AVASCULAR NECROSIS OF THE CAPITULUM OF THE ELBOW

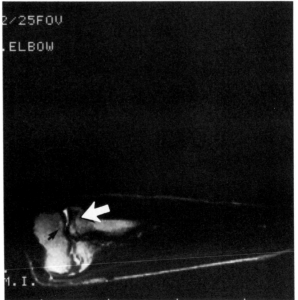

Figure 1 demonstrates the characteristic irregular signal loss in the capitulum adjoining the articular surface of the elbow. The curved white arrow demonstrates the humeral shaft for orientation. The large arrow points to the radius, and the small arrow designates the area of avascular necrosis. The changes are similar to those seen in the hip. The only true difference is the location and the bone. This avascular necrosis of the capitulum is known as *Panner's disease*.

Figure 2 is an axial orientation. The long-stemmed arrow demonstrates another view of the avascular necrosis. Note the fairly well-circumscribed sclerotic decreased signal along the articular surface. The large arrow points to the radial shaft. Figure 3 is a T2-weighted consecutive axial image again demonstrating the altered signal of the bone at this level. The small arrow points to the radial head on Figure 3a. The large white arrow points to the radial head on Figure 3b.

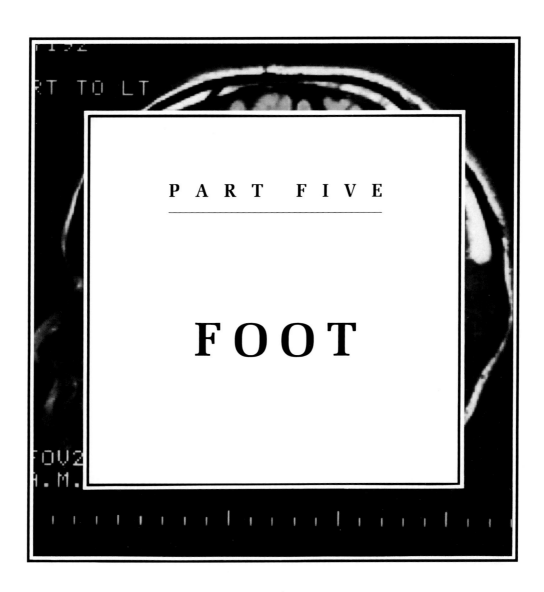

PART FIVE

FOOT

5.1 ANEURYSMAL BONE CYST OF THE CALCANEUS

A fairly well-demarcated cystic structure arising from the midportion of the calcaneal bone is identified (large arrow, Figure 1). Some central content of low signal is seen (small arrow). The axial image (Figure 2) again verifies the cystic appearance, with the large and small arrows again denoting a central structure that represents either a free-floating bone fragment or an old retractile clot. Figure 3 is a coronal image through the lesion. A simple or hemorrhagic cyst cannot be excluded from the differential diagnosis. This mass does not have features that suggest malignancy. The possibility of an intraosseous lipoma was raised in the initial discussion; however, the signal's characteristics demonstrate a signal increase more marked than that of the fat of the subcutaneous tissues in the ankle adjacent to the calcaneus. Blood can give a more profound or increased signal, as can some collections of a very high-protein fluid. This is somewhat helpful in discounting lipoma as the first differential choice, although it cannot be totally excluded. Incidentally, note how well the morphology of the ankle mortise and talar is demonstrated. There is also a nice demonstration, particularly in the sagittal plane, of the subtalar aspects of the hind foot.

This case is through the courtesy of Dr. Robert Chiteman of Maryland Magnetic Imaging.

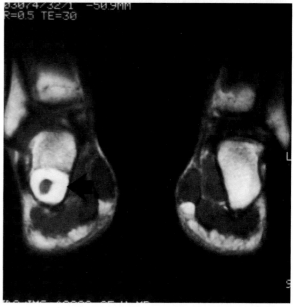

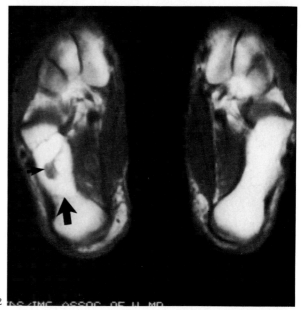

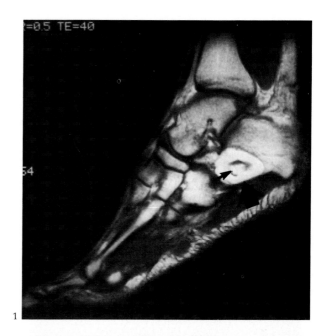

173

5.2 PARTIAL ACHILLES TENDON TEAR

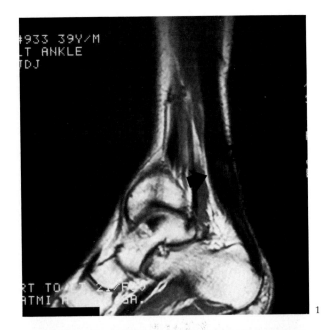

1

This 39-year-old male had an abrupt injury to the Achilles tendon. Figure 1 demonstrates, instead of the normal low signal, discrete Achilles tendon widening and a central area of increased signal (curved arrow). The large arrow points to the expanded Achilles tendon. Figures 2 and 3 demonstrate on the left (curved arrow) the diffuse increase in the tendon, in contrast to the normal right Achilles tendon (short arrow). Various tendons and ligaments are easily investigated, particularly with the improving surface coil technology. Although the clinical history and physical exam make diagnosis of many of these structures quite easy, for purposes of documentation the MRI scan offers a dramatic visual record.

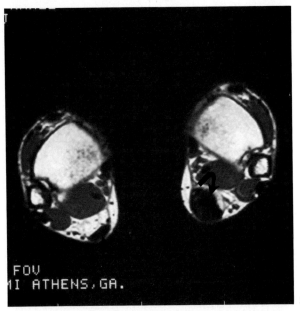

2

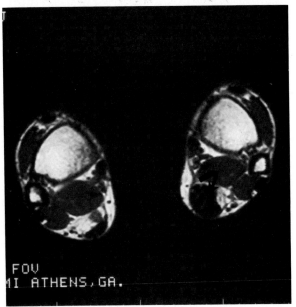

3

5.3 TALAR AVASCULAR NECROSIS

This is a 23-year-old male with previous trauma to the ankle. Figure 1 demonstrates the characteristic signal loss throughout the talus of avascular necrosis. Figure 2 (large arrow) demonstrates, in the coronal plane, the loss of signal in the talar bone. The avascular necrosis is also demonstrated in the axial plane on Figure 3 (curved arrow). Contrast this to the normal bright signal of the normal intramedullary marrow on the right side (open arrow).

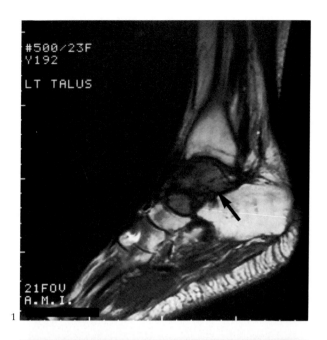

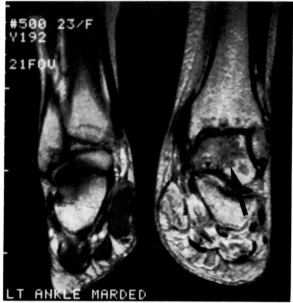

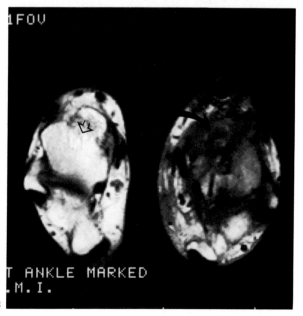

5.4 FRACTURE OF THE HEAD OF THE METATARSAL BONE

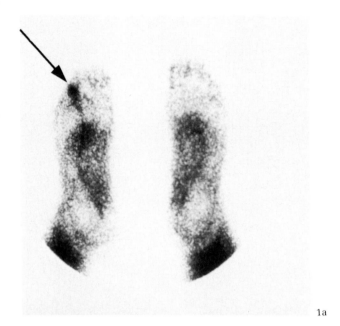

1a

1b

This is a 31-year-old male who has undergone an extensive workup that included a nuclear medicine scan (Figure 1a), as well as a CT scan to evaluate pain in the metatarsal head. Plain films (Figure 1b) demonstrate no evidence of an apparent fracture. There was a clinical interval in following this patient. However, an MRI scan was ordered, which demonstrated (Figures 2a and 3) a fracture through the head of the metatarsal (curved arrows). Figure 2b (straight arrow) is an axial cut through the fracture site. Although fractures are usually not difficult to work up, the persistence of pain, as demonstrated here, sometimes makes extensive workup in an extremity frustrating. MRI is uniquely sensitive to early changes in bone marrow and cortex secondary to fracture and can be used as an investigative tool when routine, less costly, and less involved procedures fail to yield a satisfactory answer.

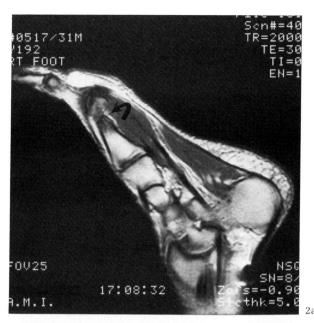

2a

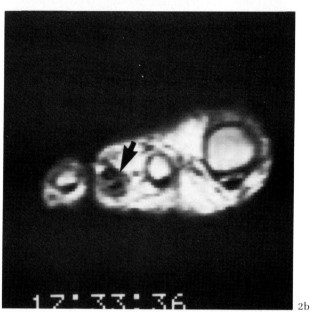

2b

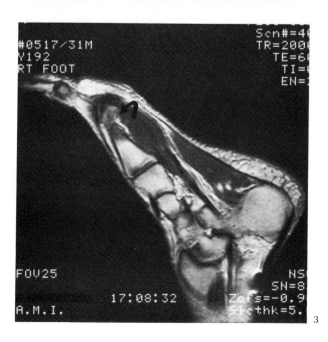

3

177

5.5 ACHILLES TENDON DISRUPTION

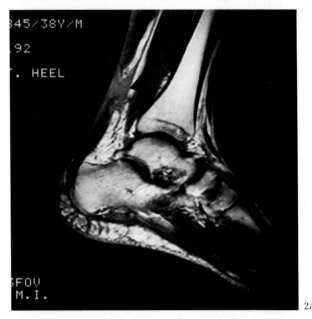

2a

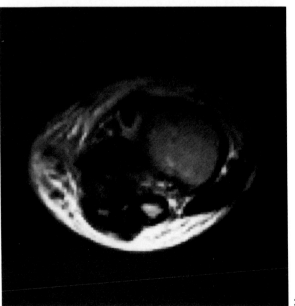

2b

Figure 1 demonstrates hematoma and edema at the site of the totally disrupted Achilles tendon. The level of disruption is at the musculotendinous interface. The more distal tendon is intact and can be followed into its insertion into the calcaneus. Figure 2a also demonstrates the area of disruption in another cut from the same sagittal series (large arrows). Note that the tendon toward the calcaneus is more normal in its appearance, with a low-signal, well-demonstrated structure. The insertion site of the calcaneus can also be identified. The damage to the associated muscle can also be followed superiorly. Figure 2b demonstrates the distorted appearance of the tendon; some of the more viable strands are still seen floating within a sea of edema and hemorrhage. Figure 3a demonstrates a slightly different level, the intact tendon going toward the calcaneal bone (curved arrow).

Figure 3b demonstrates, in the coronal plane, the area of tearing (curved arrow).

The most informative orientation is a sagittal view demonstrating the Achilles tendon. Axial scans help confirm the situation and provide additional information. For most traumatic orthopedic work, a good proton balance or T1-weighted image that enhances the anatomy is our preferred investigative tool. The differential inflammatory changes contrast sharply to the normal subcutaneous tissues surrounding the structures of the extremity. T1- and T2-weighted series are more helpful in diagnosing infection and neoplasm. When given a history of trauma, our goal is to visualize the damaged structures optimally in the most informative orientation. MRI, particularly in the sagittal and coronal planes, can also help some surgeons stage repair of various types of damage to ligaments or tendons if this is appropriate.

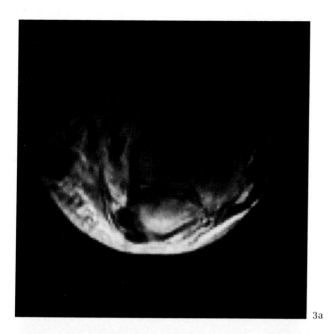

3a

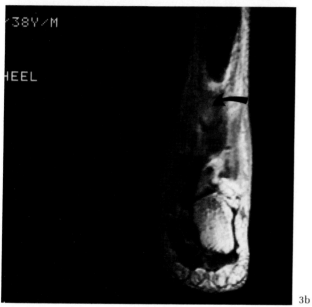

38Y/M

HEEL

3b

179

5.6 CALCANEAL FRACTURE

This patient had continued pain in the foot and a history of trauma. Figure 1 demonstrates a disruption of the cortex and a fracture line extending through the lateral aspect of the calcaneus (open arrow). In addition, there is soft tissue swelling adjacent to the calcaneus (curved arrow). Figure 2 again demonstrates the fracture line. Note that the fragment is not displaced, and despite attempts to evaluate this calcaneus by plain films, no fracture was documented. This area of disruption correlated closely with the clinical presentation of pain in this region. Note that there is again a small amount of soft tissue edema between the outer cortex of the calcaneus and the peroneus tendons.

5.7 BONE INFARCTION IN THE TIBIA

This is a 21-year-old male with a painful ankle. Figure 1, a sagittal image, demonstrates the characteristic fairly well-circumscribed, low-signal rim and high-signal center of a bone infarction. There is no suggestion of a matrix. The altered signal around the infarct can be contrasted to that of the normal bone marrow-containing regions. Figure 2 is another cut from the sagittal images demonstrating again the low-signal rim. Figure 3 is a coronal cut through the same area of infarction. Bone infarctions, particularly old ones, are sometimes difficult to differentiate from enchrondromas on plain films. However, with MRI, there is no demonstrable matrix in this lesion. This is characteristic of a simple bone infarction.

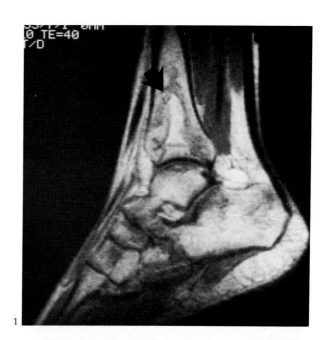

1

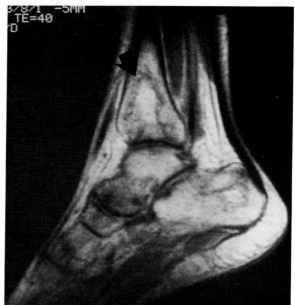

2

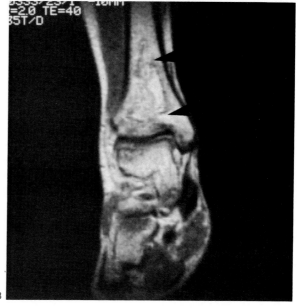

3

5.8 DELTOID LIGAMENT DAMAGE

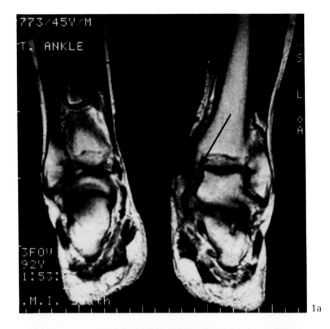

1a

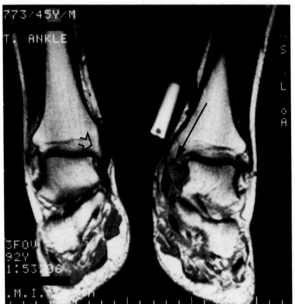

1b

The medial ligament complex on the left ankle has been torn (Figure 1a, long-stemmed arrow). Figure 1b demonstrates the intact normal right deltoid ligament (open arrow), in contrast to a slightly different level coronal view through the torn and damaged medial ankle ligament or the deltoid ligament complex. The water bottle seen in this image is used to locate the area of clinical concern, as well as to avoid confusing the left and right sides, particularly when patients may be inserted in a nonorthodox fashion into the gantry for scanning of body parts other than the routine spine, head, or body coil orientations. Figure 2a is a more confusing sagittal image, but it demonstrates the surrounding edema and the inflammatory reaction. The arrow points to the diffuse sheet-like appearance of the edema, which is intermediate in signal; contrast this to the surrounding subcutaneous fat. Figure 2b is a coronal image, which is I feel more useful in this particular case for visualization of the deltoid ligament (small arrow). Note the absence on the left side of a normal low-signal band like the one seen on the right at this same level on an axial cut (Figure 3). The sheet-like area of intermediate signal reflects altered water content secondary to edema surrounding the ligament. This secondary sign of edema can be very helpful in treating partial tears, sprains, or chronic trauma to a ligament.

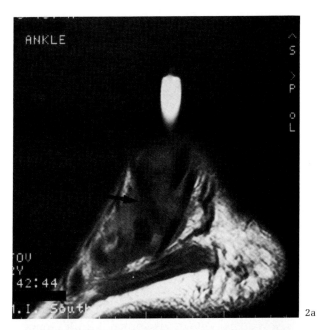

2a

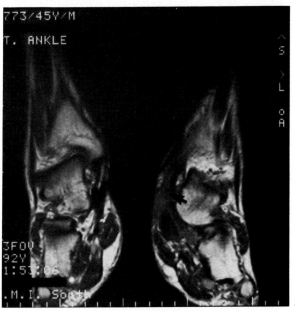

2b

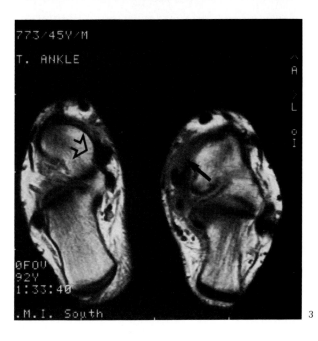

3

183

5.9 REPAIRED ACHILLES TENDON

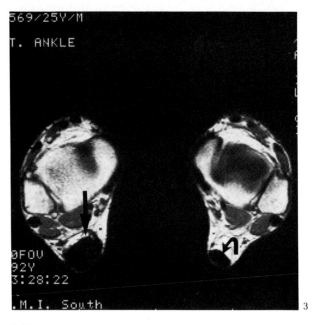

This is a previously disrupted Achilles tendon. Figure 1, a sagittal view, demonstrates the somewhat thickened, abnormal appearance of the tendon. Note that the surrounding subcutaneous tissues now maintain a normal high signal. Figure 2 demonstrates, in a slightly different sagittal cut of the same acquisition, the appearance of a thickened, slightly bulky Achilles tendon.

Figure 3 is an axial cut that again confirms the bulky, abnormally large appearance of the now repaired tendon. Contrast this to the left side (curved arrow). Note the discrete, small, low signal seen in the normal Achilles tendon.

The ability of MRI to demonstrate the edema surrounding to a ligament repair can help to determine whether the repair has failed or whether there is continued inflammation at the site of prior damage. There is some difficulty because, particularly with chronic trauma, fibrosis can mimic edema surrounding an ankle. The more chronic the damage, the closer the clinical correlation needed, particularly with studies of the extremities.

5.10 DISRUPTED ACHILLES TENDON

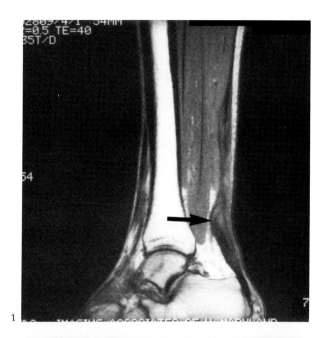

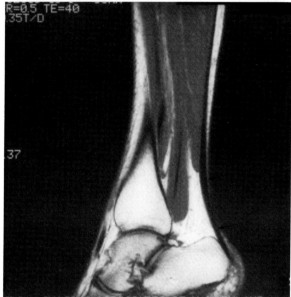

Figure 1 demonstrates distortion of the Achilles tendon secondary to trauma. Compare this to Figure 2 (small arrows). Traumatic disruption of the Achilles tendon is a fairly straightforward clinical diagnosis. However, the ease of visualization does allow documentation of the extent of the damage and differentiation between a complete disruption and a partial disruption of the Achilles tendon. The axial images (Figures 3a and 3b) demonstrate, at slightly different levels, the alteration of the normal low-signal, well-defined Achilles tendon (small arrow), in contrast to the traumatized Achilles tendon on the right (large arrow).

This case is through the courtesy of Dr. Robert Chiteman of Maryland Magnetic Imaging.

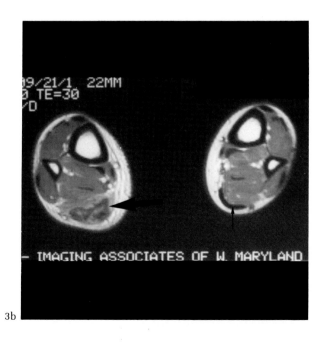

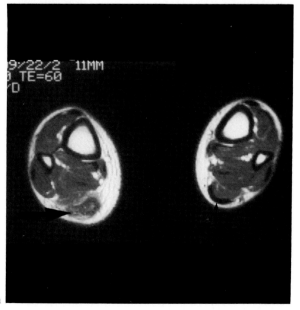

5.11 OSTEOARTHRITIS OF THE FIRST METATARSAL

Figure 1a (curved arrow) demonstrates the normal osteophytic prolific change in the joint between the metatarsal head and the proximal phalanx. Figure 1b demonstrates the lipping of the osteophyte (open arrow). Figure 2 demonstrates the axial cuts through the normal cortex and the intramedullary content of the adjacent metatarsal versus the osteoarthritic metatarsal head.

Although this diagnosis by plain film is satisfactorily evaluated, it is interesting to observe the precursor to the plain film finding of bone, that is, the erosion of the articular cartilage and the narrowing of the joint space that lead to the secondary reaction of bone in the form of an osteophytic formation. I would not advocate the use of MRI for a diagnosis of osteoarthritis, particularly at this later stage. However, in the early stages, MRI is an excellent investigative tool for evaluating the hyaline cartilage of articular surfaces in helping to delineate at-risk patients with arthritis.

Figures 3a and 3b demonstrate enhancement of a small amount of effusion within the joint affected by the osteoarthritis.

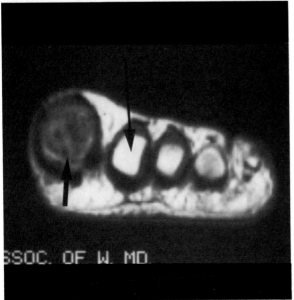

1a

1b

2

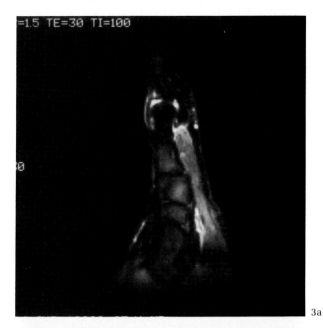

3a

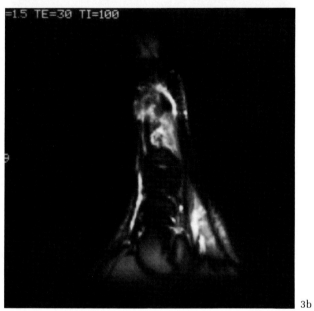

3b

187

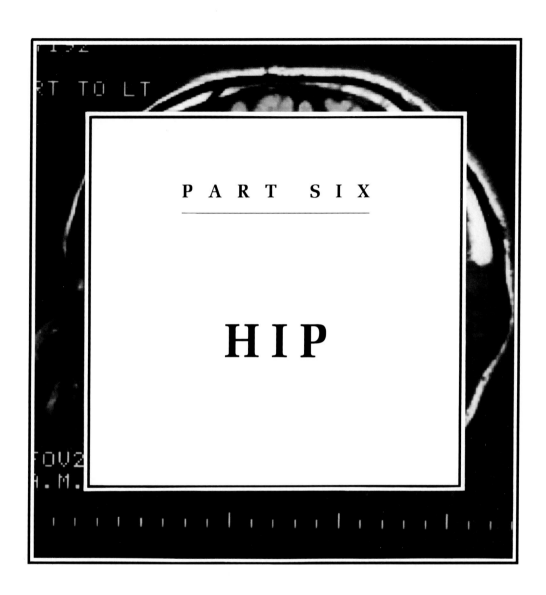

PART SIX

HIP

6.1 METASTATIC DEPOSIT IN THE LEFT FEMORAL HEAD

Figures 1a and 1b demonstrate a characteristic metastatic lesion within the left femoral head (solid arrow). On Figure 1b there is a small superior area of normal signal in the femoral head. It would be a highly unusual for an avascular necrotic process to spare the weight-bearing surface. In addition, there is thinning and what appears to be cortical destruction along the more lateral uncovered area of the femoral head (Figure 1a). Figures 2 and 3, which are axial images, also demonstrate the characteristic low-signal appearance of the metastatic disease, as well as thinning and probably destruction of the cortex, particularly in the posterior aspect of the humeral head (large arrows). Contrast this to the normal appearance of the right femoral head.

Figure 2 (small arrow) points to a small area of preserved normal signal within the left femoral head.

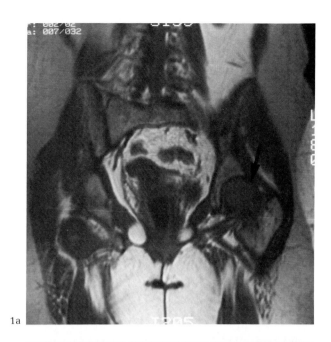

1a

1b

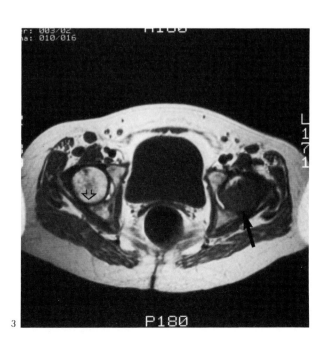

3

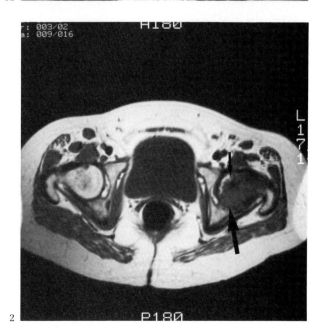

2

6.2 AVASCULAR NECROSIS OF THE LEFT HIP

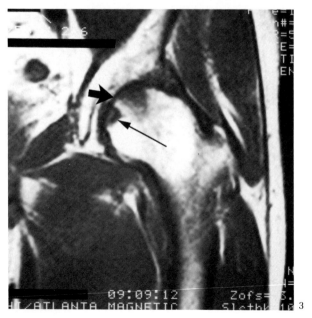

This 65-year-old male had a painful hip that has worsened in the past 3 years. A wedge-shaped area of decreased signal is nicely identified on the coronal image (Figure 1, large solid arrow).

The axial image on Figure 2 also demonstrates this wedge-shaped area of low signal consistent with avascular necrosis.

Figure 3 is a zoom-up view of Figure 1 demonstrating the normal ligamentum teres (long-stemmed arrow) adjacent to the characteristic avascular necrosis-type lesion (solid arrow). The ligamentum teres should not be easily confused with avascular necrosis. The rim is usually much better defined, and the ligamentum teres in its characteristic lateral position is usually separate from the more weight-bearing surface of the femoral head, although some avascular necrosis can be seen in this area.

6.3 BILATERAL AVASCULAR NECROSIS

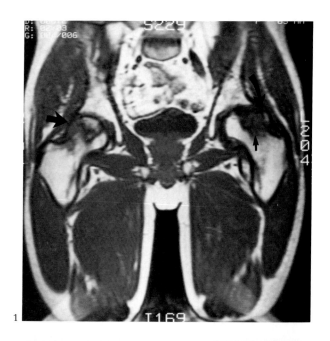

1

Figure 1 demonstrates typical late manifestations of avascular necrosis. There is a diffuse vascular area of low signal involving the femoral head on the left. There is also remodeling and flattening of the contour of the femoral head. Contrast this to the appearance of the plain film (Figure 2, large arrows).

The right side of the femoral head has also undergone fairly advanced avascular necrosis-type changes (large solid arrow). The femoral head maintains its normal contour; this can be confirmed on the plain film (Figure 2).

Figure 3 is an axial cut through the involved femoral heads.

Figure 4 demonstrates the flattening of the femoral head (arrows) on the left side. Also note the presence of joint effusion in both hips (curved arrows).

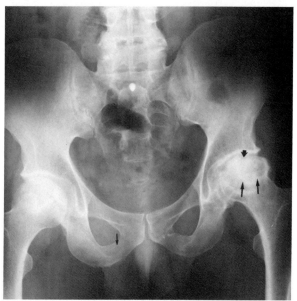

2

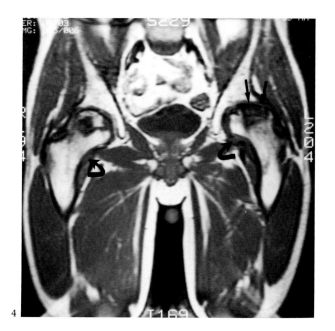

4

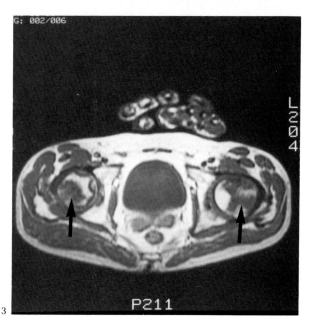

3

6.4 EARLY AVASCULAR NECROSIS OF THE LEFT HIP

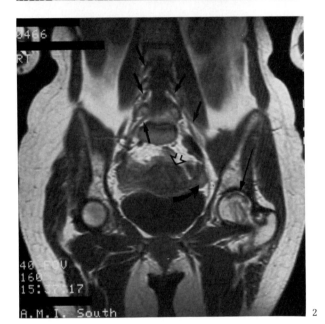

Figure 1 demonstrates a small focal area of decreased signal along the weight-bearing surface of the left femoral head (long-stemmed arrow). Contrast this to the normal high signal of the uninvolved right femoral head (arrowhead). This particular cut also demonstrates the ability of the MRI body coil coronals to demonstrate the normal pelvic viscera, such as the uterus, and the endometrial lining denotes the lumen (open arrow).

Additional structures of note are the exiting nerve roots (arrows) from the lumbosacral spine.

Figure 2 is a slightly more anterior cut demonstrating the well-circumscribed, low-density ring and a more high-signal central area of involved bone (long-stemmed arrow).

Again, note the exiting nerve roots from the lumbar thecal sac (small solid arrows). The uterus is again identified (open arrowhead). The adnexal structures, including the fallopian tubes and ovaries, can also be visualized and inspected (solid curved arrow).

Figures 3a and 3b demonstrate, in the axial plane, the appearance of this avascular necrosis. This example shows the necrosis involving the more posterior aspect of the femoral head; however, the characteristic low-signal ring involvement, a vascular distribution, and an area of weight-bearing articular surface are key features of the typical avascular necrosis. The relationship of the bladder, rectum, and uterus is well defined on this axial cut, as it is on the CT scan of the pelvis (open arrowhead).

The importance of visualization of the normal pelvic viscera, particularly in the workup of hip and back pain, cannot be underestimated. This is particularly true in females if the routine lumbar investigation has failed to delineate a significant disc abnormality to explain radiating sciatic or hip pain and body coil imaging for avascular necrosis has proven unsuccessful. The explanation is often a pelvic mass, which can be evaluated at the same time as the hip. We have found various cancers and benign masses to be the cause of radiculopathy. Orthopedic surgeons now use a pelvic CT or MRI scan if the more routine investigation of the lumbar spine and hip region with MRI is not satisfactory to explain a patient's complaint.

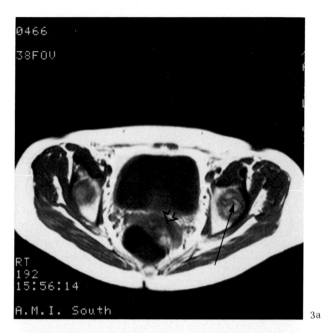

3a

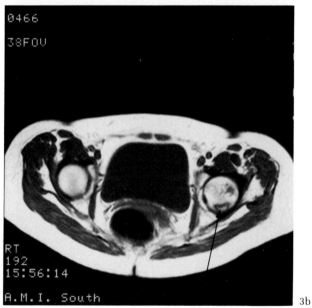

3b

195

6.5 MILD AVASCULAR NECROSIS

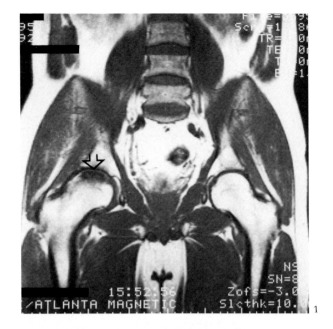

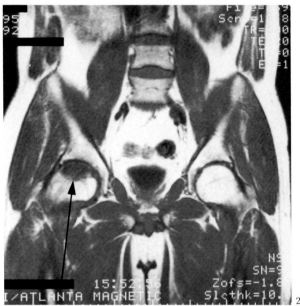

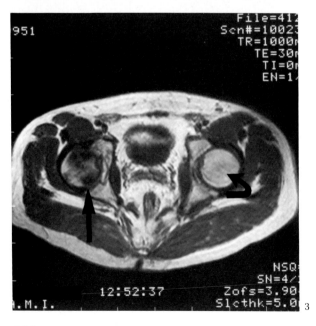

Figures 1 and 2 demonstrate a focal diffuse area of decreased signal intensity. This is a later stage of avascular necrosis than avascular necrosis with a ring and a high-signal center. Note, however, that the femoral head (Figure 1, open arrowhead) still maintains its normal anatomic contour. Figure 2 demonstrates the vascular wedge-like pattern involving the weight-bearing surface (long-stemmed arrow).

Figure 3 is an axial cut through the involved right femoral head. Note the demonstration of low signal in the area of involvement. Contrast this to the normal left hip (curved arrow).

6.6 BILATERAL AVASCULAR NECROSIS

Figure 1 demonstrates the geographic ring in the weight-bearing surface, with a vascular distribution in both the right and left hips (long-stemmed arrows). The changes are characteristic of an avascular necrosis. Bilateral involvement is not unusual.

Figures 2 and 3 are axial cuts through the involved femoral heads. In this particular case, no joint effusion is identified. The femoral heads maintain their normal contour. The neck and shafts also maintain their normal signal.

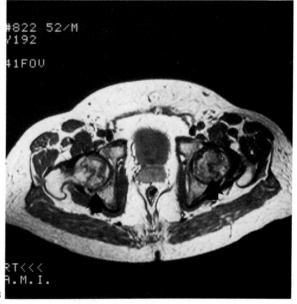

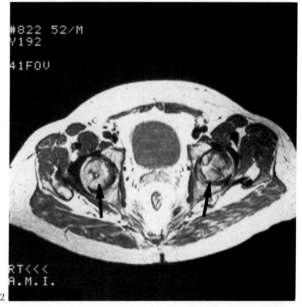

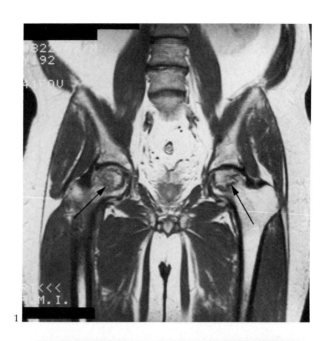

197

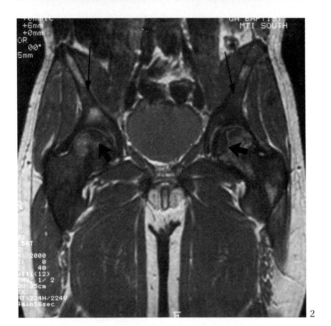

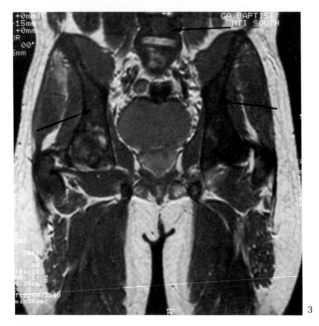

6.7 AVASCULAR NECROSIS IN A PATIENT WITH SICKLE CELL ANEMIA

Figure 1 (arrows) demonstrates characteristic areas of signal void; this is consistent with avascular necrosis along the weight-bearing surfaces and in the articular region of the femoral heads (large arrows). Note also that there is decreased signal and patchy areas throughout the bone marrow-containing spaces, representing a return to a more hypercellular, hematopoietic bone marrow. This reflects the increased need for production of red blood cells in a patient with sickle cell anemia.

Figure 2 again demonstrates the areas of avascular necrosis, which can be very difficult to differentiate, particularly in a patient with diffuse infiltrating bone matter change, as seen here. The only real clues are the abutment of the area up to the articular surface, the wedge-shaped vascular pattern, and the location and characteristic decrease in signal, which is slightly more than that of the other areas of hypercellular infiltration.

Also note on Figure 3, a slightly more posterior cut, is the hypercellular appearance of the large portion of the bone marrow (long-stemmed arrows). The vertebral bodies, which represent a significant area of hematopoiesis in the body, also reflect the return of the bone marrow to a more hypercellular state. Some patchy areas of more increased signal, which represents a more typical partially fatty bone marrow, can be identified in the bony structures on all three images.

6.8 AVASCULAR NECROSIS SECONDARY TO STEROID USE IN A PATIENT WITH LEUKEMIA

This 15-year-old male has developed fairly severe avascular necrosis (large arrow, Figure 1). There is signal loss, as well as flattening and remodeling of the femoral head on the left. The changes extend throughout the epiphysis down to the epiphyseal plate. The normal appearance of the epiphysis on the right is identified. The epiphyseal plate can also be easily identified (open arrow).

Figure 2 is an additional cut through the avascular necrosis centrally. In this area, there is a slight increase in signal. Various patterns and stages of avascular necrosis have been well described. It is usually well circumscribed, always occurs on a weight-bearing surface, and produces a vascular pattern.

Figure 3 is an axial cut demonstrating the normal right femoral head in the axial plane (open arrow). Contrast this to the geographic area of decreased signal rim with a more high-signal center (curved white arrow).

The appearance of avascular necrosis with chronic steroid use is well documented. MRI increases the ability to detect the changes of avascular necrosis, hopefully at an earlier stage, allowing possible modification of steroid use; however, in a patient with leukemia, management choices are limited. Early detection may allow a central orthopedic coring procedure. The appearance of flattening of the femoral head, however, changes the grading, as well as the orthopedic management.

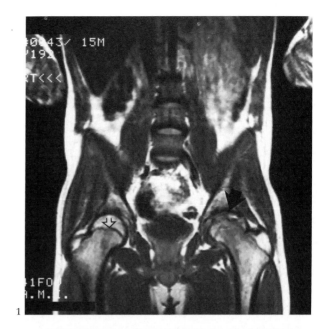

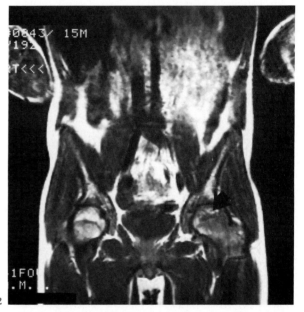

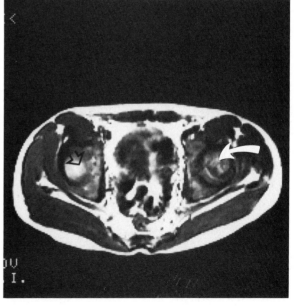

6.9 SEVERE OSTEOARTHRITIS OF THE LEFT HIP WITH EFFUSION AND GEODE FORMATION

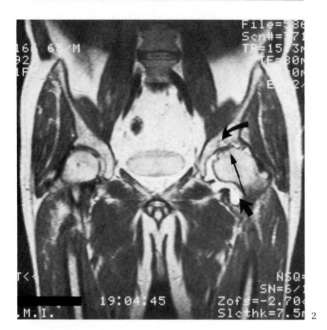

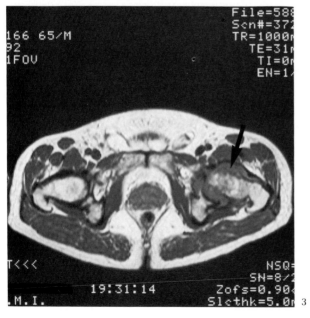

Figure 1 demonstrates narrowing of the more lateral weight-bearing surface of the left hip with maintenance of normal signal in the femoral head (long-stemmed arrow). This is associated with a fairly large joint effusion (large solid arrow). A subchondral cyst or geode is evident in the roof of the acetabular fossa (curved arrow).

Figure 2, a T2-weighted image, demonstrates increased signal of the joint effusion (long-stemmed arrow). Note the absence of any focal signal loss in the weight-bearing portion of the femoral head, the degenerative lateral osteophytic spurring of the acetabular roof, and the formation of the geode containing some fluid, which is also enhancing (curved arrow).

Figure 3 is an axial cut again demonstrating the large size of the joint effusion.

The features seen are typical of an osteoarthritic change within the hip. Joint effusion is not unusual in these areas. The reaction of bony spurring along the lateral acetabulum should also be considered characteristic of an osteoarthritic hip.

The early damage, however, involves the highland cartilaginous surface. Cracks in the surface allow transmission of fluid, which can form small cysts or pockets deep to the subchondral bone, resulting in geodes (Figure 3, arrow).

6.10 BILATERAL AVASCULAR NECROSIS WITH EFFUSIONS

This is a 35-year-old male complaining of bilateral hip pain. The changes of focal decreased signal in the weight-bearing portion of the femur have been clearly established as representing avascular necrosis.

Figure 1 demonstrates the typical low signal encountered in the hip (large arrows). This is easily contrasted to the rather high signal from the normal marrow in the lower portion of the femur and the iliac bone. The contour of the femoral head can also be evaluated in regard to any loss of the normal contour or presence of flattening of the head. The orthopedic surgeon will use the findings of avascular necrosis, with or without femoral head flattening, to guide the therapeutic decision. A nondeformed head allows a coring procedure to be attempted in hopes of revascularizing the femoral head and avoiding an implant procedure. In this case, the right femoral head appears to be slightly flattened.

The presence of effusion can be seen with avascular necrosis. The effusion is seen in Figure 2 as high signal with a T2-weighted image. However, even the T1-weighted image (Figure 3) can demonstrate the effusion (open arrows).

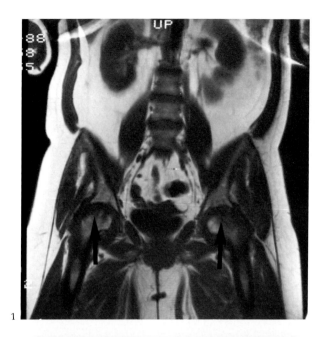

1

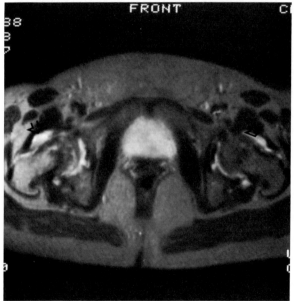

2

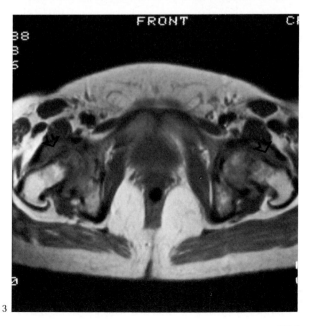

3

6.11 SEVERE DEGENERATIVE JOINT DISEASE AND EFFUSION

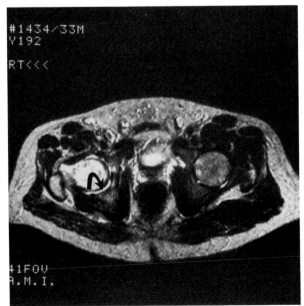

This is a 33-year-old male with evidence of marked narrowing of the joint space of the right hip (arrow, Figure 1). Note that the femoral head has been flattened.

Figure 2 demonstrates an attempt to remodel the lateral roof of the acetabular fossa (large arrow). There is also evidence of joint effusion (small arrow).

Figure 3a demonstrates distention of the joint capsule secondary to joint effusion (arrows). Figure 3b is a T2-weighted image demonstrating increased signal in the joint effusion (curved arrow).

This represents a severe degenerative change without avascular necrosis. This patient's hip had been traumatized in the past, which allowed early, severe osteoarthritis. The images, however, allow exclusion of avascular necrosis.

The presence of effusion can be seen in severe osteoarthritis; however, based on MRI criteria alone, it is difficult to exclude the possibility that the effusion itself may be infected. However, we can exclude underlying osteomyelitis from the bony structures with a high degree of confidence.

Septic effusions tend to erode rapidly the cortical bone in the joint. As with plain films, this may be a key feature allowing exclusion of a septic arthritis within a joint space.

6.12 DIFFERENT STAGES OF BILATERAL AVASCULAR NECROSIS

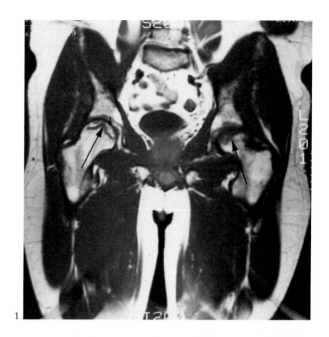

Figure 1 demonstrates the focal signal loss diffusely through a weight-bearing surface on the left, in contrast to the low-signal ring and high-signal center on the right.

This reflects the earlier and later stages of avascular necrosis. Ischemia causes death of the cells within the marrow, as well as osteocyte formation. Eventually, an attempt is made to revascularize the area with mesenchymal cells and capillaries permeating the necrotic segment. This is the later stage seen on the left side in Figures 1 and 2. The high-signal center seen on the right represents necrotic bone that has not yet been revascularized.

Figure 3 consists of axial cuts through the avascular necrosis on both sides, again demonstrating the ring and high-signal, nonrevascularized bone on the right (the small arrow points to the high-signal necrotic focus, and the long-stemmed arrow points to the low-signal ring).

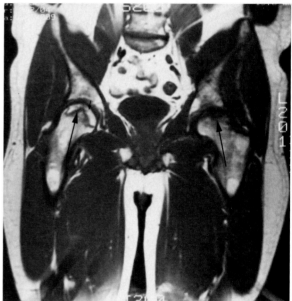

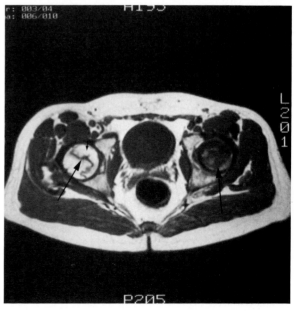

6.13 SACRAL METASTATIC INVOLVEMENT

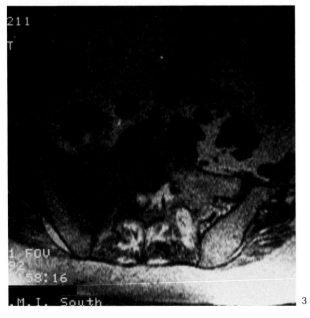

This is a patient with a known primary cancer and pain in the pelvic and sacroiliac regions. Figure 1 (large arrow) demonstrates the characteristic signal loss in the right sacral region that abuts but does not extend into the sacroiliac joint. There is also some extraosseous soft tissue extension into the neuroforaminal canal (long-stemmed arrow).

Figure 2 demonstrates (curved arrow) the extension of the extraosseous soft tissue into the neuroforaminal canal (curved arrow). Note that this displaces the sacroiliac nerve route to the left (arrowhead). The characteristic signal loss on the right (arrowhead) can be contrasted to the normal appearance of the sacral bone on the left.

Figure 3 again demonstrates signal loss in the same patient. Note that the abnormal bone changes are arrested at the sacroiliac joint. Also note that the changes do extend into the sacral vertebral body (large arrow).

6.14 RIGHT AVASCULAR NECROSIS WITH LONG-TERM STEROID USE

This is a 51-year-old male with a 10-year history of steroid use demonstrating characteristic signal loss in the anterior weight-bearing surface of the right femoral head (see Figures 1a and 1b, large arrows). Figure 2 is an axial cut demonstrating the anterior location of the geographic well-circumscribed area of altered signal. Figure 3 (arrow) is a sagittal cut through the area of avascular necrosis. The typical altered signal is easily identified on the coronal and axial images and easily contrasted to the normal left side. The geographic loss of signal, which fits a very vascular pattern, is also easily identified and reproduced on typical images of avascular necrosis. The predilection for the weight-bearing surface is also characteristic and allows a differentiation between this abnormal ischemic state and that of metastatic disease, which can have a very similar low-signal appearance.

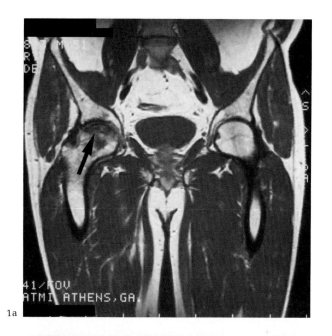

1a

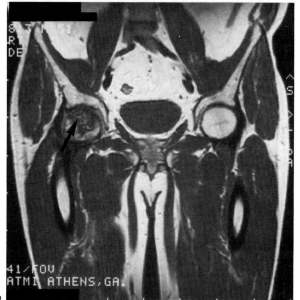

1b

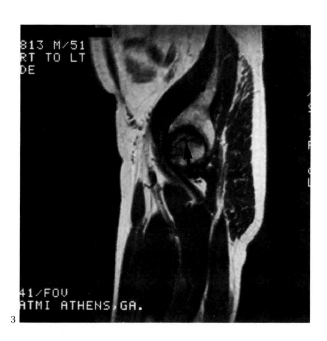

3

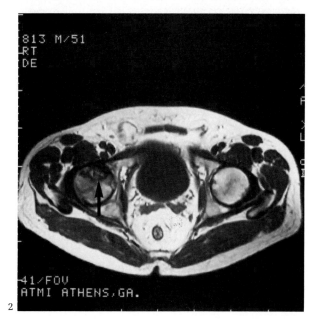

2

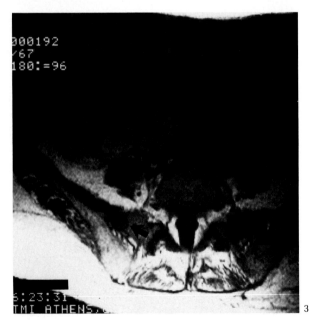

6.15 ADENOPATHY AND BONY METASTATIC INVOLVEMENT IN THE PELVIC REGION

Figure 1 demonstrates the loss of the normally easily identified aorta (arrow) and inferior vena cava (arrowhead) secondary to the surrounding of the vessels by adenopathy (curved arrows).

Figure 2 demonstrates additional nodes at a slightly different level of the axial series (large arrow). These nodes are intermediate to slightly higher in signal than the psoas muscle. The same criteria used with CT, that is, exclusion of the normal vessels, allows any other rounded retroperitoneal mass to be viewed with suspicion as possibly representing a metastatic adenopathy.

Figure 3 demonstrates an association with the adenopathy (large arrow). There is a focal decrease in signal in the sacrum consistent with metastatic bone invasion (short arrows).

It is usually incidental to a routine lumbar spine, but the retroperitoneum is also clearly evaluated and should always be inspected in patients with back pain to exclude aneurysm, metastatic disease, or adenopathy.

6.16 BILATERAL AVASCULAR NECROSIS WITH EFFUSIONS

Figure 1 demonstrates typical signal loss in the weight-bearing surfaces of the femoral heads (arrows). Effusion is also present (long-stemmed arrow). Figure 2 is a slightly different cut from this coronal series again demonstrating the loss of normal signal in the weight-bearing surface consistent with avascular necrosis (arrows). The joint effusion on the right can also be easily documented (long-stemmed arrow). Figures 3a and 3b are axial cuts through the femoral heads demonstrating the presence of avascular necrosis, which is clearly demarcated from the normal signal of the spared femoral head (arrows).

Also note that effusions are present bilaterally. This is a typical associated finding of avascular necrosis (long-stemmed arrows).

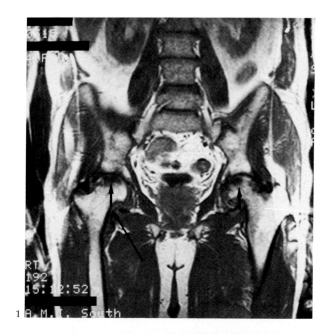

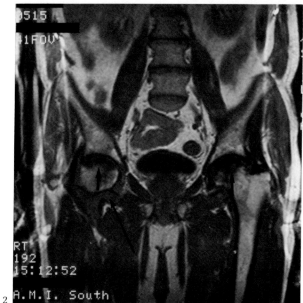

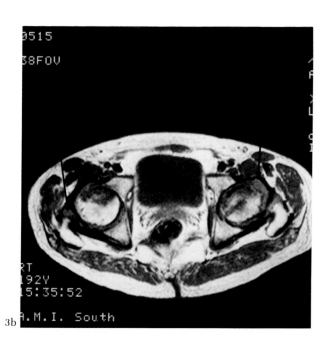

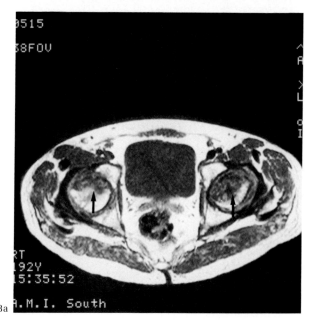

6.17 LEFT AVASCULAR NECROSIS WITH FEMORAL HEAD FLATTENING

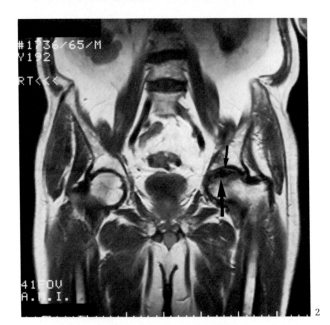

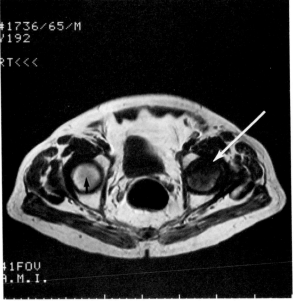

Figures 1 and 2 demonstrate the late changes of avascular necrosis in the left hip. The focal area of low signal in the weight-bearing surface is identified (large arrow). Also note that the femoral head has lost its contour and collapsed. This is the result of the trabecula compromise secondary to cellular ischemia, causing the trabeculae to collapse upon themselves. It is also the result of compression of the trabeculae, as well as the increased cellularity secondary to ischemic debris. Attempts at revascularization are also responsible for the absence of or decrease in signal in the weight-bearing area.

Figure 3 is an axial cut through the avascularly involved left femoral head (long-stemmed white arrow). This involves predominantly the more anterior portion of the femoral head. In this example there is some alteration of signal in the more posterior head, suggesting that the vascular damage may not be as complete here; however, this may also reflect the more preferential collapse of the femoral head anteriorly. Contrast this to the normal-appearing right femoral head (small arrow).

6.18 CHANGES OF MULTIPLE MYELOMA IN THE PELVIC BONES

This 64-year-old male with proven multiple myeloma demonstrates the diffuse, infiltrative hypercellularity of the bone marrow. Figure 1 demonstrates the altered low signal of the left femoral head, neck, and shaft (curved arrow). Contrast this to the spared, more normal marrow in the femoral head on the right (arrowhead).

Figure 2 demonstrates the diffuse involvement throughout the neck and shaft on the left and right (large arrow). This same diffuse, infiltrative pattern can be identified in the vertebral bodies (open arrow).

Figure 3 consists of axial cuts through the hips. The open arrows point to the relatively normal, more fatty marrow that is still present on the right side, involving a portion of the femoral head and the greater trochanter.

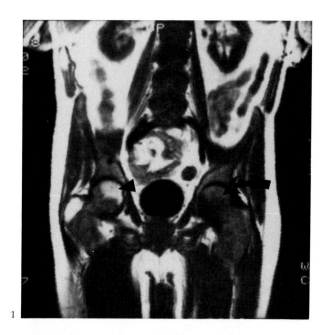

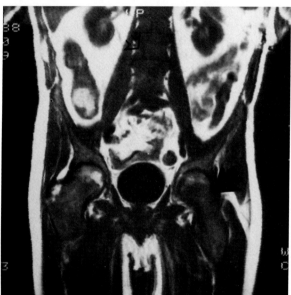

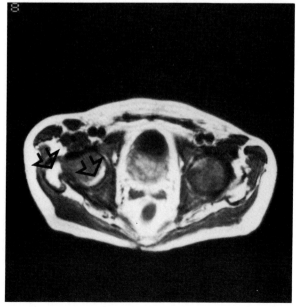

6.19 BILATERAL AVASCULAR NECROSIS

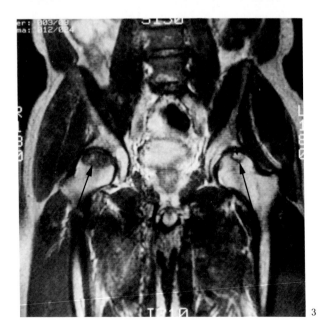

This is a 58-year-old male with bilateral avascular necrosis. The larger area of more long-standing involvement is seen on the right (long-stemmed arrow). The left femoral head also demonstrates a focus of avascular necrosis in a more early stage. Note the high-signal center and low-signal ring (arrows). The essential signal characteristics of the more T1-weighted image of Figure 1, the proton density image of Figure 2, and the T2-weighted images of Figure 3 remain fairly constant and reflect predominantly signal loss in the area of avascular necrosis.

Figure 4 demonstrates the changes in the axial plane (arrows). The short arrow shows a high-signal center with a low-signal ring seen with the earlier changes of avascular necrosis.

Trauma, alcohol abuse, and steroid therapy are the most common causes of avascular necrosis, although certain blood dyscrasias that cause thickening or increased viscosity of the blood are also associated with this disorder.

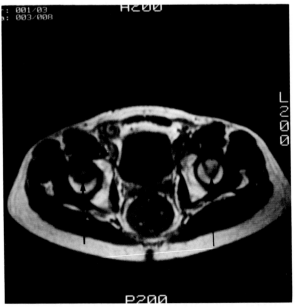

6.20 EFFUSION OF THE RIGHT HIP

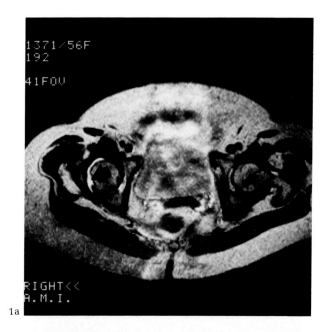
1a

This is a 56-year-old female with a nonspecific effusion. MRI is very sensitive to the presence of even scant amounts of fluid within the joint space (Figures 1a and 1b, arrow).

The coronal images on Figures 2 and 3 also demonstrate the ease of visualization of small amounts of effusion in the coronal plane.

The cortical bone can be inspected. The bone marrow and trabeculae can also be inspected, allowing exclusion of metastasis or underlying infection. MRI is sensitive to early bone marrow changes that reflect metastasis, infection, and vascular change. It is also quite sensitive to the presence of small amounts of effusion, which may herald arthritis or joint infection.

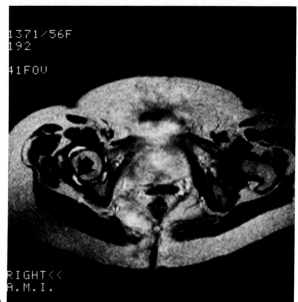
1b

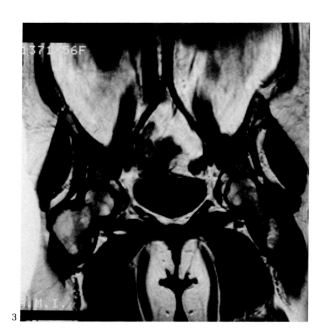
3

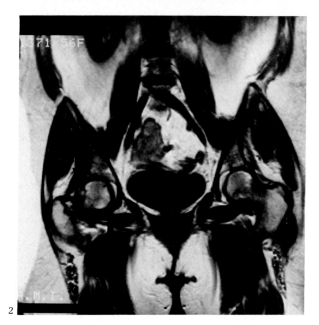
2

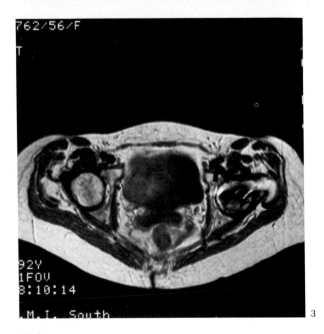

6.21 AVASCULAR NECROSIS IN THE PRESENCE OF A HIP PIN

This 56-year-old female had hip pinning for a fractured femoral neck. There is continued left hip pain.

Despite the metallic artifact (large solid arrow, Figure 1), there is good detail of the more superior weight-bearing bone, which shows loss of signal consistent with avascular necrosis (curved arrow). This can be compared to the normal right hip (open arrow). Figure 2, which consists of axial cuts through the normal right hip (arrow), demonstrates a metallic artifact, as well as some visualization of surrounding bone (curved arrow).

Figure 3 demonstrates again the separation of the fairly normal image immediately around the periphery of the metal pin (curved arrows).

It is always worthwhile, even when a metal prosthesis is in place, to attempt to image a body part if the information will be helpful to the patient. Surprisingly, an abundance of information is available, and the artifact, although present, is minimized by the ability to scan through the body part in more than one plane. In CT scanning, star artifact tends to be heavier and degrades the image more thoroughly than MRI. MRI provides the ability to "look around" the artifact and see the necessary anatomy.

6.22 LUMBAR AND PELVIC METS

This is a 65-year-old male with nonspecific hip and back pain. Figures 1a and 1b demonstrate extraosseous extension of tumor arising from the inferior aspect of the greater tuberosity of the left femur (large arrow). Note the extraosseous extension into the soft tissues (small arrow). In addition, the diagnosis of metastasis is confirmed by the visualization of a large paraspinal mass arising from the right lower lumbar paraspinal region (curved arrows).

Figures 2 and 3 also demonstrate the disruption of the cortex and the altered signal in the bone in the greater tuberosity (large arrows). The extent of involvement can be followed fairly accurately and delineated from the more normal appearance of bone (arrowheads).

On the right, the arrowheads (Figure 2) demonstrate a small amount of effusion in the right hip, which is a much less specific finding.

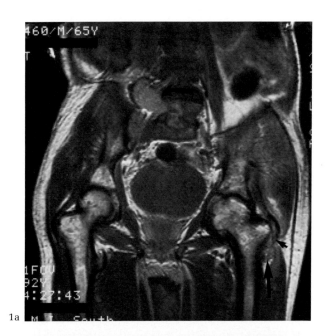

1a

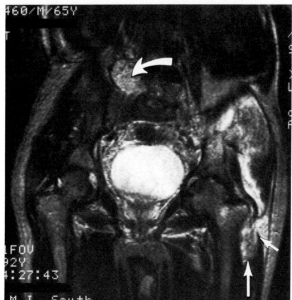

1b

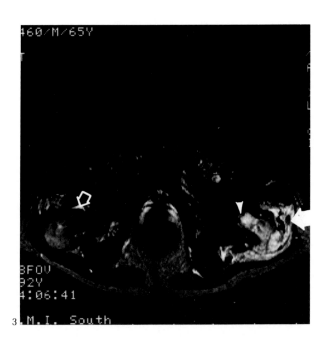

3

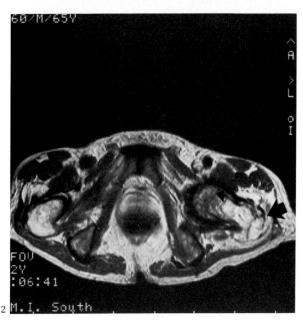

2

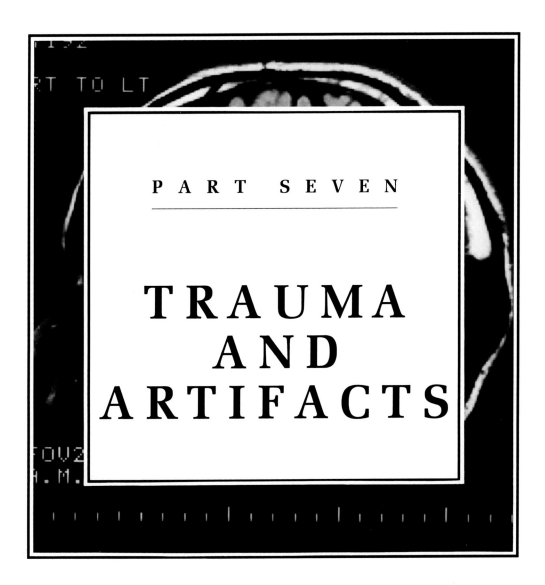

PART SEVEN

TRAUMA
AND
ARTIFACTS

7.1 OLD HEALED FIBULAR FRACTURE

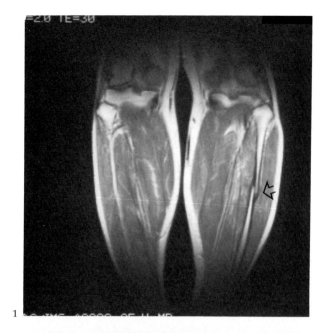

1

Figure 1 demonstrates overlap of fracture fragments, and the open arrow points to the fracture site. Note that the cortex of the fracture region has been fused. There is normal signal within the intramedullary portion of the fractured fibula, and the surrounding soft tissues are also normal.

Figure 2 is a sagittal cut again demonstrating the overlapping of the fracture fragments and the normal appearance of the fused cortex following healing (small arrows). Figures 3 and 4 are T1- and T2-weighted axial cuts through the fracture area. Note that the intramedullary canal maintains a normal high signal consistent with normal marrow, and the cortex shows the homogeneous low signal. There is no alteration or evidence of extraosseous material to suggest neoplastic change underlying the obvious fracture.

MRI is definitely excessive for evaluation of routine fractures. However, in some patients, the lack of any significant trauma raises the possibility of underlying bone abnormality to explain the fracture. MRI is an excellent investigative tool to exclude a diffuse infiltrating process, which may not be detectable on the basis of plain film alone.

This case is through the courtesy of Dr. Robert Chiteman of Maryland Magnetic Imaging.

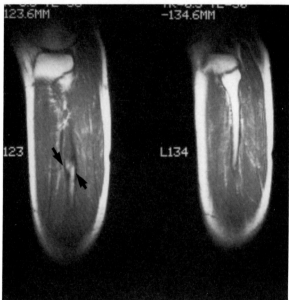

2

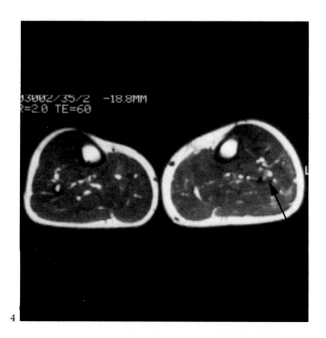

4

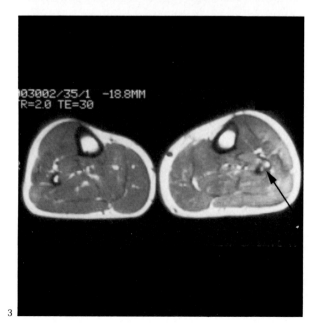

3

7.2 RECTUS MUSCLE HEMATOMA WITH FOLLOW-UP STUDY

This is a 17-year-old male. Figure 1 demonstrates the altered signal of the inferior surface of the rectus femoris muscle (large arrow). Figure 2 is a proton density-weighted image demonstrating the fairly well-defined hematoma. At this point, the hematoma is subacute and demonstrates a homogeneous high signal. Contrast this to the normal rectus muscle on the left (curved arrow). Figure 3 is a T2-weighted image again demonstrating the high signal, which exceeds that of the surrounding fat (straight arrow). Contrast this again to the rectus muscle on the left, which is normal (curved arrow).

Figures 4 to 6 are studies done approximately 6 weeks following the first study. They demonstrate contraction of the hematoma and narrow, small, low-signal ring (arrow). Again contrast this to the left rectus muscle on the left (curved arrow). Figure 4 is a T1-weighted image. Figure 5 is a proton or a mixed weighted image, and Figure 6 is a T2-weighted image. The involution of a mass helps in differentiating between hematoma and lipoma. However, with a good history and the signal characteristics, lipoma should be easily excluded from the differential alternatives.

This case is through the courtesy of Dr. Rodolfo A. Lopez and Dr. Paul Griffin of Pasadena Magnetic Imaging.

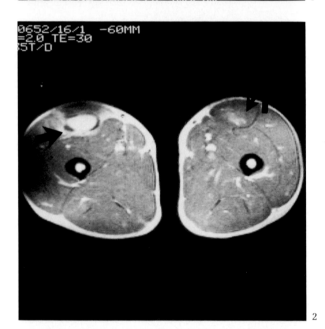

1

2

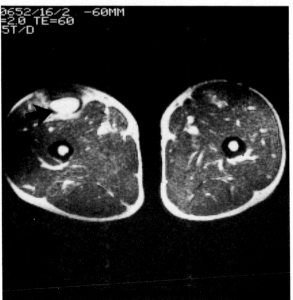

3

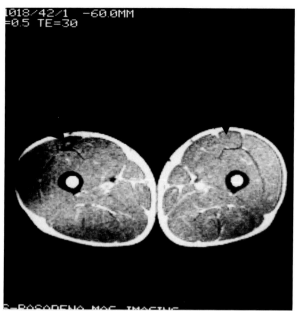

4

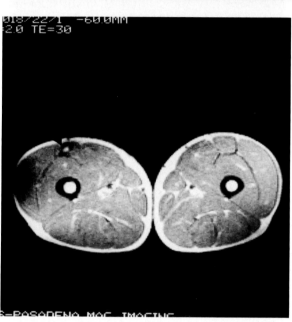

5

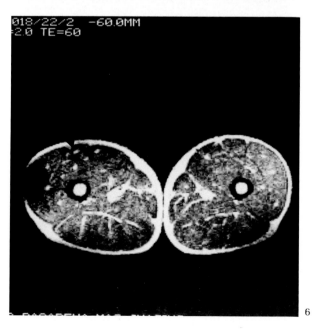

6

219

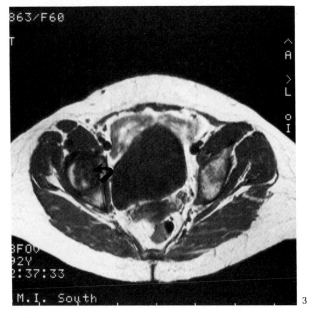

7.3 OLD FEMORAL FRACTURE INCIDENTAL TO HIP WORKUP FOR AVASCULAR NECROSIS

Figures 1 and 2 demonstrate the distorted and overlapping shaft of the fractured left femur (large arrow). Note the fusion of the cortex and the periosteal remodeling of this fracture, which is now quite old.

Incidental note is made of the typical signal loss in the weight-bearing area of the hip on the right side (curved arrow). This is consistent with avascular necrosis (Figures 1 and 3).

The ability to image the cortical line as well as the intramedullary region allows some assessment of cortical and periosteal new bone formation, although plain films are still believed to be most sensitive in showing deposition and normal bone formation following a fracture. This case is included because of its nice demonstration of the relationship of the fracture fragment and the new cortex remodeling. It also demonstrates that the intramedullary content can be visualized and abnormal fracture can be excluded.

7.4 C5–6 OLD FLEXION-ROTATION INJURY

Figures 1a and 1b demonstrate anterior flexion of the C5 on 6 vertebral bodies. Note the anterior offset (small arrow) and the undisturbed cord (large arrow).

Most interesting on the MRI scan is the demonstration in the parasagittal cut (Figure 2) of the subluxed and perched facet at C5–6 (long arrow). The facets almost always are nicely demonstrated on a cervical study, and the parasagittal cuts are very informative in regard to the alignment of the facets. Figure 3 shows the offset of the vertebral body C5 (large arrow), demonstrating the end plate, and small arrows demonstrate the end plate of C6. Note the slightly rotated appearance of the cord.

The use of numerous images without manipulating the spinal column is particularly advantageous in the acutely traumatized patient.

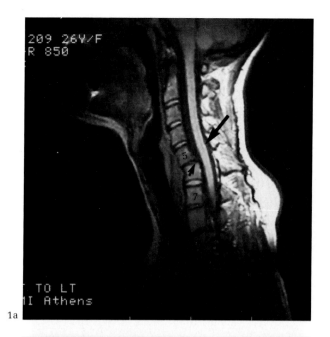

1a

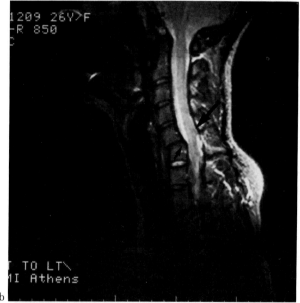

1b

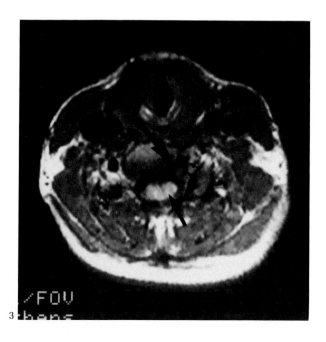

3

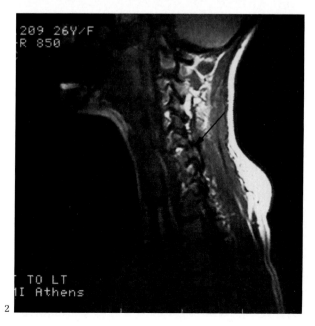

2

221

7.5 VARICOSITIES AND SUBCUTANEOUS EDEMA

This is a 29-year-old female with clinically evident varicosities. Figure 1 demonstrates the tortuous superficial veins (long-stemmed arrow). Figures 2 and 3 demonstrate in the coronal view numerous dilated veins within the subcutaneous tissues. The MRI imaging of such a condition is usually not applicable to a clinical setting. This case is used simply to demonstrate the prominent appearance of the varicosities. These should not be confused with other subcutaneous dermal lesions.

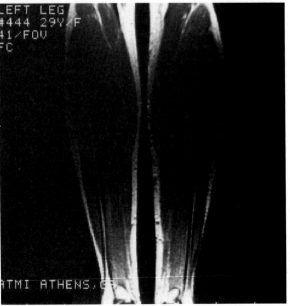

7.6 FLEXION FRACTURE IN THE CERVICAL REGION

Figure 1 demonstrates at C5 compression secondary to flexion deformity following a motor vehicle accident. The solid arrow demonstrates the slightly deformed and compressed vertebral body. Note that there is a decrease in the overall signal representing compression of the bony trabecula, as well as edema, which decreases the signal in the marrow-containing compartments. The open arrow demonstrates traumatic herniation of soft tissue posterior to the C5–6 disc space.

Figure 2 is a T1-weighted scout film demonstrating similar findings. The elevation of the posterior annulus designated by the open arrow also helps confirm the presence of traumatic herniation.

Figure 3 is an axial cut through the C5–6 level that demonstrates, slightly less dramatically, the presence of the herniation. Note the ease of relating the herniated material and the deformed vertebral body to the cord and the ability to inspect the cord for intrinsic damage.

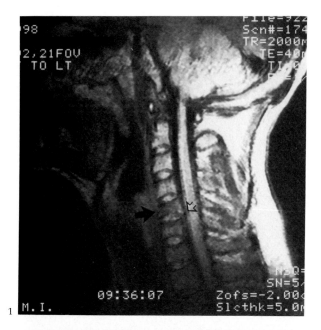

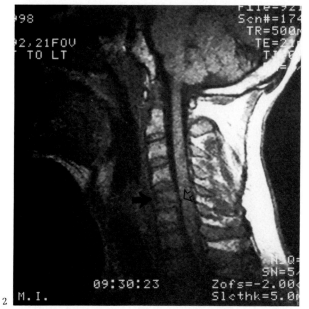

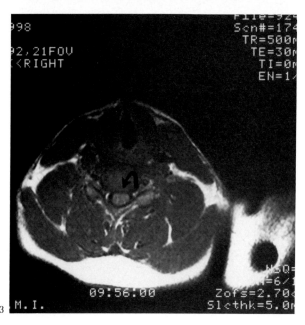

7.7 MILD COMPRESSION DEFORMITY OF THE L3 VERTEBRAL BODY

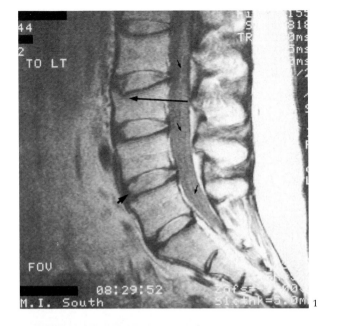

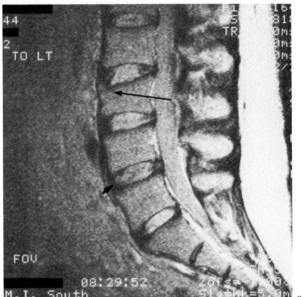

Figure 1 demonstrates compression of the end plate of L3 (long-stemmed arrow). Note the downward slope of the compressed end plate. Contrast this to the normal intervertebral disc and the superior end plate (small arrow). Tiny arrows demonstrate the ability to see the nerve roots as they pass through the thecal sac.

Figure 2 is a T2-weighted image again demonstrating the mild compression deformity of the L3 vertebral body. Note that despite trauma, this particular disc maintains a relatively normal signal. This is contrasted to the slight degenerative change noted at the L4–5 level. Usually a small amount of compression at a disc level will be associated with accelerated degenerative changes at this level. However, this is not constant and needs to be described for evaluation of discogenic pain in relation to remote injury to the vertebral column.

7.8 CORD ATROPHY SECONDARY TO TRAUMA WITH VERTEBRAL KYPHOSIS SECONDARY TO COMPRESSION FRACTURE

Figure 1 demonstrates the apex of a kyphotic angulation secondary to compression fracture. The large arrow point to the now wedged, chronically compressed and deformed vertebral bodies. The open arrow demonstrates a cord of normal length superior to the area of bony damage. Figure 2 is a zoom-up view of the same sagittal image. The arrows delineate a slightly small, stretched, and attenuated cord at this level, representing atrophic cord as it is stretched and compromised over the apex of the kyphosis at the T11–12 level.

Figure 3 demonstrates the neuroforminal canals (arrows). Note that the exiting nerves can be identified within the canals.

The ease of MRI, and imaging both the neurologic structure and the associated bony deformity secondary to trauma, allows MRI to be a primary investigative tool, as well as an excellent way to follow up for additional damage to the cord and for additional loss of stature with remodeling of the vertebral column.

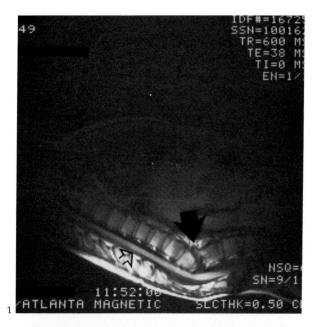

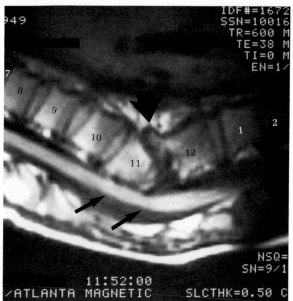

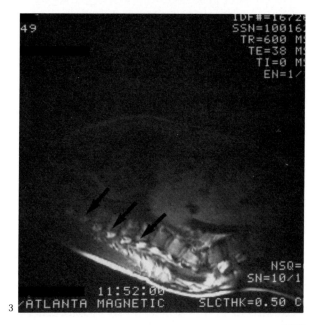

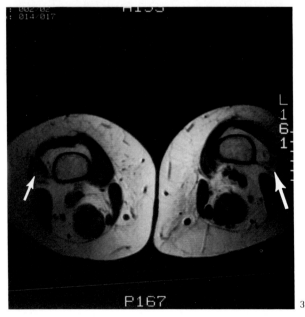

7.9 VASTUS LATERALIS MUSCLE WITH FATTY CHANGES SECONDARY TO DISEASE

The patient has undergone placement of implants in the left knee. In Figure 1, the normal vastus lateralis seen on the right demonstrates the intermediate signal of healthy muscle. Contrast this to the signal on the left (curved arrows); the arrowhead demonstrates the medial extent of the now fatty-like muscle. Figures 2 and 3 demonstrate again in the axial plane the absence of normal intermediate signal in the vastus lateralis on two contiguous sections. The small arrow points to the normal vastus lateralis muscle. The large arrow points to the fatty muscle in the vastus lateralis. This can be easily contrasted to the more normal muscle in the left thigh. Views of the other extremity are usually very helpful for additional comparison. Disuse or neurogenic interruption of innervation to the muscle can result in fairly homogeneous fatty replacement. This can be differentiated from neoplasm by the absence of any increase in the size of the area of abnormal signal.

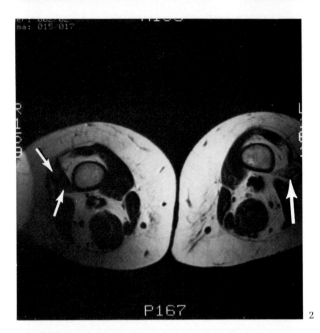

7.10 RUPTURED ADDUCTOR MAGNUS AND SEMITENDINOSUS MUSCLE

This case demonstrates the appearance of a traumatically ruptured muscle in the thigh. The chief characteristics are the distorted and torn muscle and the redundant ligament swimming in a combination of edema and hemorrhage. Figure 1a demonstrates the axial appearance of the torn muscle. Compare this to the CT cut of Figure 1b. Very similar information is seen. However, I believe that in general the contrast of soft tissues on MRI is much higher than that of CT. The small solid arrows demonstrate the outer extent of the surrounding edema and hemorrhage. The open arrows point to the intact muscle fibers extending through the traumatically damaged region.

The sagittal image on Figure 2 demonstrates redundant tendon that has been retracted secondary to the tear into the thigh. The curved arrow demonstrates the appearance of fluid representing edema and hemorrhage; contrast this to the subcutaneous fat in other areas of the thigh. Figure 3 is a coronal image. The large arrow again demonstrates the edema and hemorrhage in this region. Up to now, a large amount of soft tissue damage has been undetected from a diagnostic standpoint. MRI offers an excellent opportunity for demonstrating torn muscle, sprained or stretched ligament, and torn ligament or tendon. Much of the disruption is clinically evident with a good history and physical exam; however, on occasion, we have an opportunity to assist the treating physician in this regard. This provides the medicolegal ability to image traumatic damage.

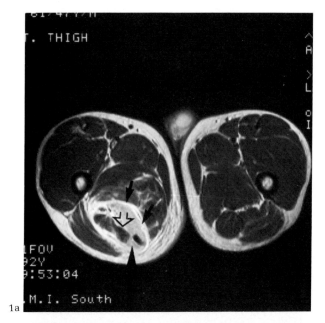

1a

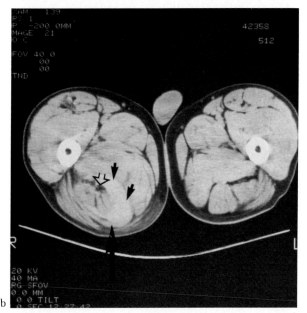

1b

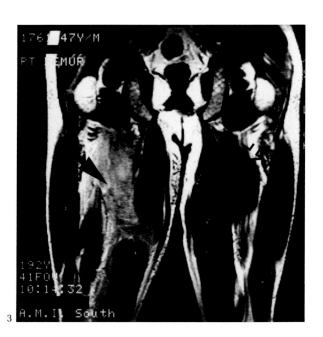

3

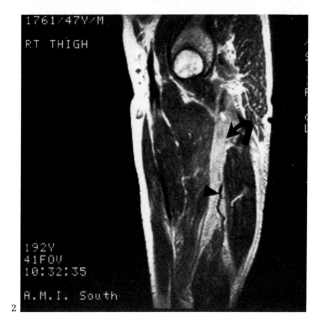

2

227

7.11 ARTIFACT FROM A KNEE PROSTHESIS

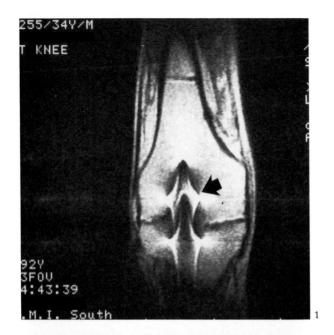

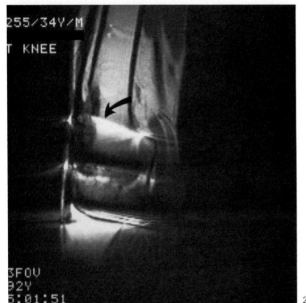

Figure 1 demonstrates field artifact through the knee in the coronal view secondary to placement of a knee prosthesis.

Figure 2 demonstrates in the sagittal plane the distortion of the image at the level of the knee prosthesis (curved arrow). It is also important to note that despite the placement of the prosthesis, the detail immediately above and below the knee joint and even some suggested detail within the knee joint is available. Aside from the well-known contraindications to the use of MRI, such as the presence of a pacemaker, aneurysm clip, spinal cord implant, and some dental and ear, nose, and throat prostheses imaging in the area of a metal implant should at least be attempted. In many cases, MRI will augment, if not surpass, any CT evaluation. The field artifact can be quite severe; however, given the multiple image orientations, they can "look around" the artifact. With CT the metal artifact usually destroys the axial images in the region of interest.

7.12 PANOPAQUE RETAINED IN THE LUMBAR SAC

Figure 1 demonstrates high signal within the thecal sac on a proton balance or slightly T1-weighted image. This maintains a fairly high signal in the T2-weighted image. Note the incidental demonstration of heavy degenerative change with loss of signal and disc alteration, as well as end plate changes (curved arrow). The arrowhead demonstrates the diffusely bulging disc. Figure 2, a T2-weighted image, again demonstrates a focus of abnormally increased signal in the lower aspect of the lumbar thecal sac (large arrow). Tiny arrows demonstrate the presence of a rootlet. The arrowhead again points to the bulging annulus, and the curved arrow again designates the heavily degenerative changes at the L3–4 level.

Figure 3 demonstrates the presence of a fluid-fluid level. This helps to confirm the suspicion that this is residual panopaque from remote myelography.

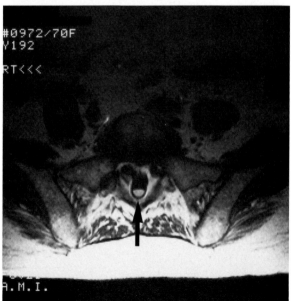

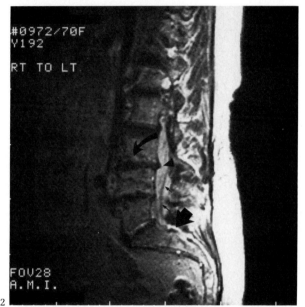

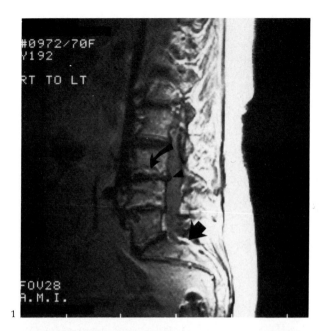

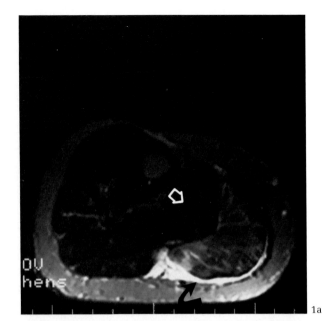
1a

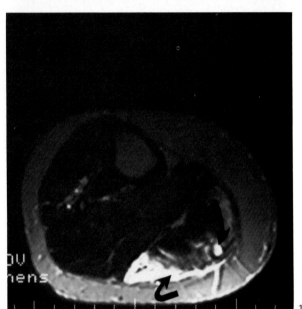
1b

7.13 RUPTURED MEDIAL HEAD OF THE GASTROCNEMIUS MUSCLE

Figure 1a demonstrates the abnormal diffuse increase in signal representing edema within the medial head of the gastrocnemius muscle (solid arrow). Contrast this to the normal surrounding muscle (open arrow). In addition, the curved arrow demonstrates a hematoma surrounding the muscle and limited by the fascial lining. Figure 1b demonstrates a small intermuscular hematoma with characteristics to those of the surrounding hematoma (curved arrow). Figure 2a demonstrates the normal left thigh and compares it to the traumatized muscle on the right (white arrow). Figure 2b is a T2-weighted image again demonstrating the altered signal and the slight increase in signal of the traumatized muscle reflecting increased water content. Also note the curvilinear area of increased signal representing a hematoma surrounding the traumatized muscle (large arrow). Figures 3a and 3b demonstrate, on the left, the normal muscle (open arrow). The large arrow points to the normal vessels coursing through the muscle mass. This is contrasted to the right side, where the irregular, torn muscle can be identified; a portion of this increase may also represent vessels passing through this area. This halo of increased signal of the surrounding hematoma can also be visualized.

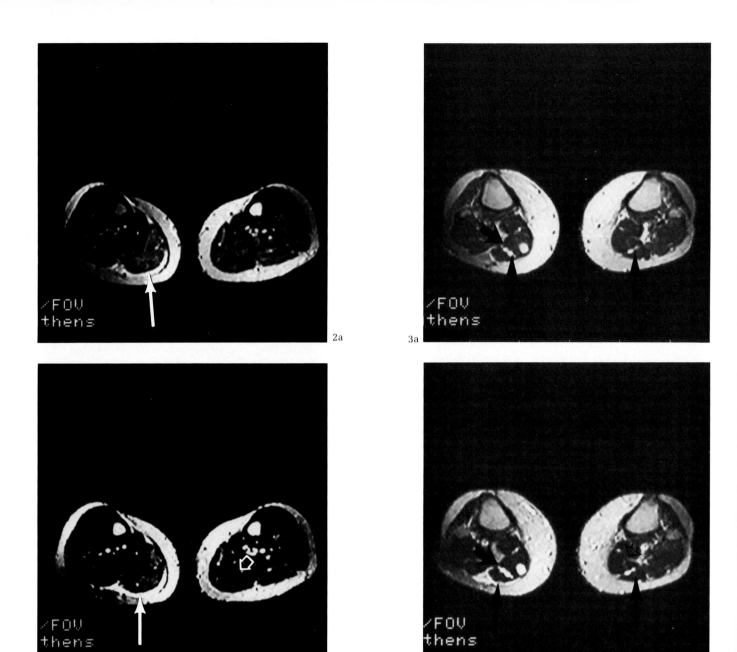

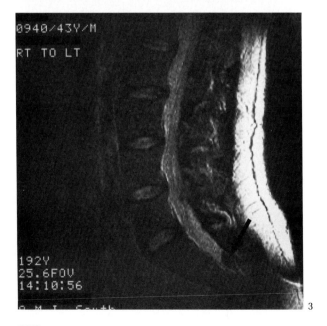

7.14 DROPLETS OF PANOPAQUE IN THE LUMBAR SAC

On the strongly T1-weighted image of Figure 1, a sagittal cut demonstrates the increased signal of the retained panopaque within the thecal sac. Note the air-fluid level (small arrow).

Figure 2 is a proton-weighted or balanced image demonstrating a slight increase in signal in the panopaque. Note that there is a slight chemical shift at the fluid-fluid interface. In the T2-weighted image on Figure 3, the panopaque now adopts a very low signal contrast to the high signal of the CSF. The axial image on Figure 4 demonstrates the fluid-fluid interface of the panopaque. We encounter a fair amount of panopaque in our middle-aged and older patients. Its presence is not a diagnostic problem; plain films help to confirm the suspicion of retained panopaque. The fluid-fluid level, its normal location, and its characteristic signal make it easy to detect and exclude it as a clinically significant finding.

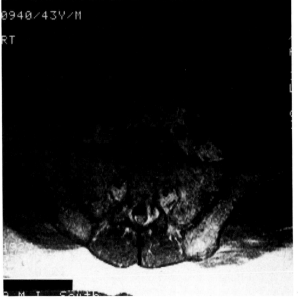

7.15 RECTUS FEMORIS TEAR AND HEMATOMA SECONDARY TO TRAUMA

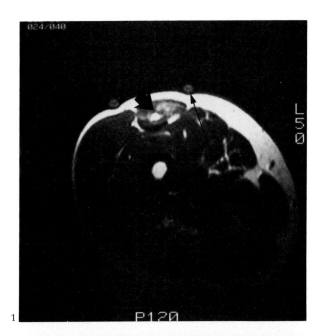

1

In this 33-year-old male, the increased signal representing edema and torn muscle fiber and the central high signal representing hematoma are identified on the axial image of Figure 1 (large arrow). The area of concern has been identified with fluid-containing vials taped over the clinically symptomatic body part (long-stemmed arrow). Figure 1 is a T2-weighted image. Figures 2a and 2b are slightly different cuts demonstrating the hematoma within the less distorted muscle fibers of the rectus femoris muscle (open arrow). Note that on the more proton density or T1-weighted images, the hematoma is less apparent; in this case, it is more accentuated by the T2-weighted imaging sequence.

Figure 3 demonstrates, less impressively, the coronal appearance of the disrupted, torn femoral muscle (solid arrow).

A history of trauma is always helpful in distinguishing clearly traumatic hematomas from lipoma or other tumors. Hematomas demonstrate paramagnetic properties seen with blood; this is usually a very homogeneous increased signal with a fairly well-defined border. Aside from the hematoma, there is no distortion of the surrounding muscle. This is usually helpful in differentiating the hematoma from a malignant muscle tumor. The signal with blood increases with the more T2-weighted parameters, whereas it is suppressed with lipomas. The surrounding subcutaneous fat can be used as a built-in monitor to help assess the fatty content within a mass to be evaluated.

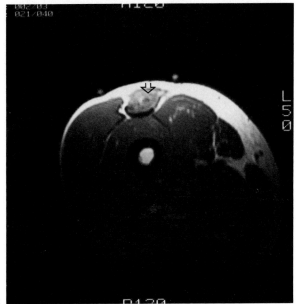

2a

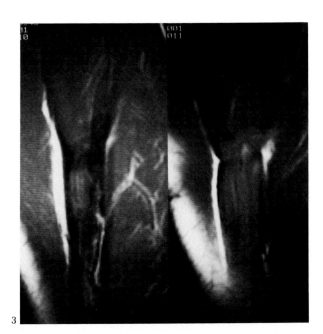

3

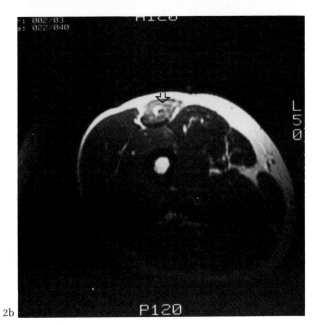

2b

233

7.16 RETAINED BULLET

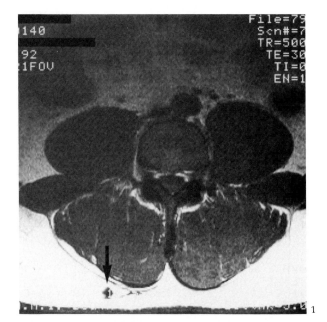

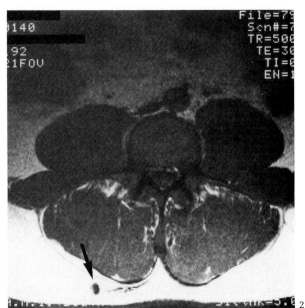

Figures 1 and 2 demonstrate the features of a metallic but nonferrous retained bullet fragment. Note the relative lack of distortion of the surrounding image.

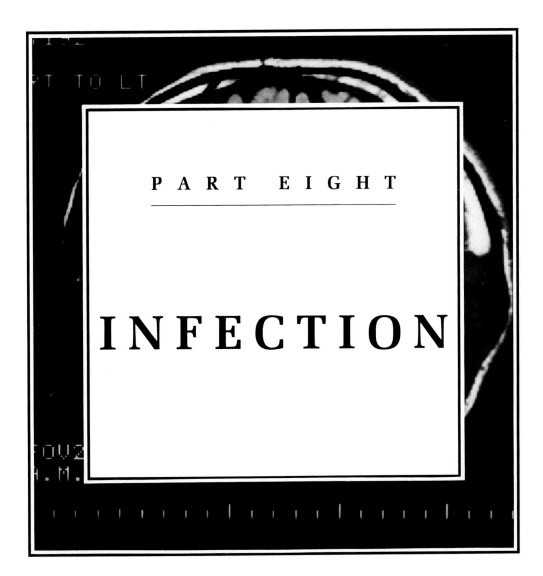

PART EIGHT

INFECTION

8.1 SEPTIC ARTHRITIS

This 70-year-old patient demonstrates the features of septic arthritis. On Figure 1, note the diffuse narrowing of the entire joint space (large arrow), as well as the decreased signal in the juxta-articular bone (open arrow). This is associated with a moderate-sized effusion. The effusion and the diffuse disruption of the cortical bone at the joint spaces (Figure 2, large arrows) allow a diagnosis of septic arthritis. However, if the patient had a history of hemophilia, hemophiliac arthropathy would be difficult to exclude.

Figure 3 is an additional sagittal cut demonstrating the effusion (curved arrow).

Also note that there is subchondral extension of fluid and inflammatory change into the tibia; this probably represents additional infection, most likely osteomyelitis. Figure 4, an axial cut, demonstrates the effusion (curved arrow), as well as narrowing of the patellofemoral articular space (arrow). Note that on all the pictures, the menisci are virtually nonexistent, having been destroyed by the inflammation and possibly by chronic trauma that may have preceded the septic arthritis.

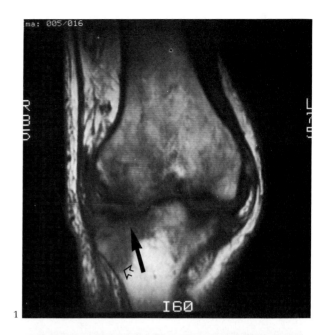

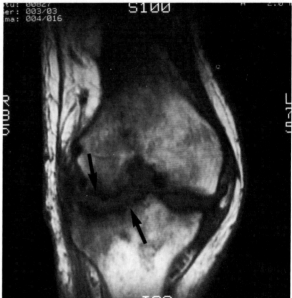

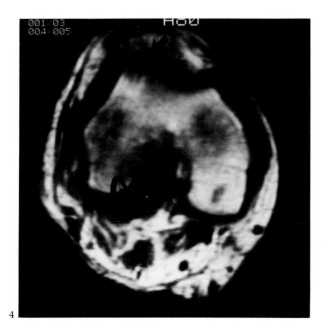

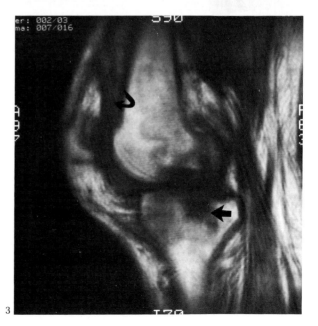

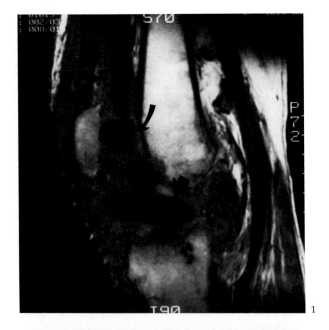

8.2 SEPTIC KNEE WITH PROSTHESIS

Figure 1 (large arrow) points to a knee prosthesis demonstrated by a diffuse low signal. Arrowheads demonstrate the presence of metal sutures. Large gas bubbles within the knee joint are identified (curved arrow). Note the large amount of effusion within the joint space (arrowheads). Figures 2 and 3 are axial cuts again demonstrating gas bubbles within the joint (large arrow). Note the diffuse amount of joint effusion (small arrows). The medium-sized arrows point to a patellar prosthesis that remains in place.

The presence of a prosthesis with gas bubbles and a large amount of effusion should suggest sepsis. The signal characteristics of effusion have a nonspecific, but abnormal character. The demonstration of gas bubbles is highly suggestive, if not pathonomonic, of inflammatory change within the fluid. Figure 4 demonstrates areas of abnormal signal within the distal shaft of the femur. The presence of a large amount of effusion, which is suspected of being septic, suggests this is a foci of osteomyelitis within the shaft itself (curved arrows).

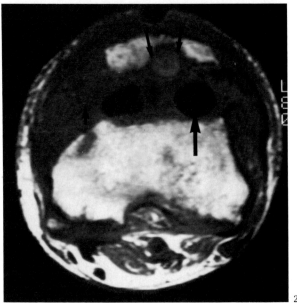

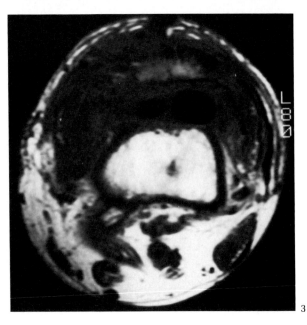

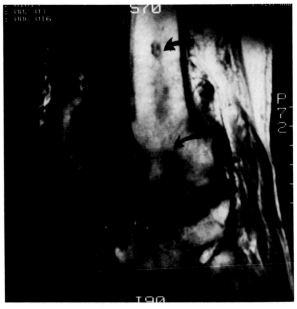

8.3 OSTEOMYELITIS OF THE DISTAL TIBIA AND TALUS

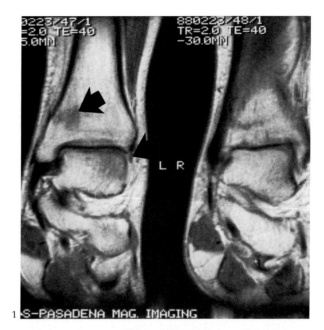

Figure 1 (large arrows) points to two fairly ill-defined areas of decreased signal in the normally high-signal bone marrow of both the tibia and the talus (large arrows). Figure 2 is a T2-weighted image demonstrating increased signal of a small joint effusion in the ankle joint. Figure 3 is an axial cut through the distal tibia demonstrating the ill-defined area of low signal within the distal tibia. This figure also demonstrates some destruction and loss of bone mineral of the cortex (open arrow).

Poorly defined areas of decreased signal represent hypercellularity or possible edema in the marrow-containing spaces. Without a clinical history, it is difficult to know definitely whether we are dealing with osteomyelitis or possible metastatic lesions. In addition, recent articles suggest that decreased signal in the bone marrow may also represent hypercellularity secondary to return of bone marrow to a erythropoietic status. Metastatic disease and red marrow reconversion would not be expected to have associated fluid. The metastatic disease alone may be suspected of eroding cortex, as seen on Figure 3. MRI is uniquely suited to demonstrating the extent of involvement and can suggest the presence of soft tissue abnormalities. However, the clinical history and physical findings are essential components in correct interpretation of the images.

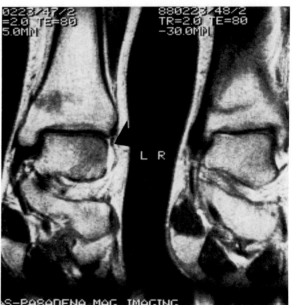

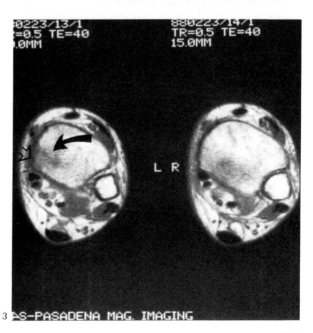

8.4 INFRAGLUTEAL ABSCESS

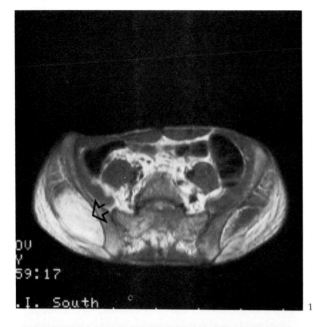

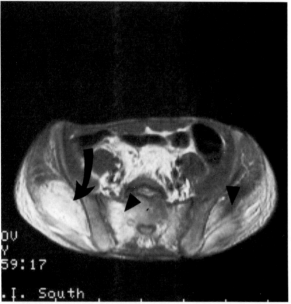

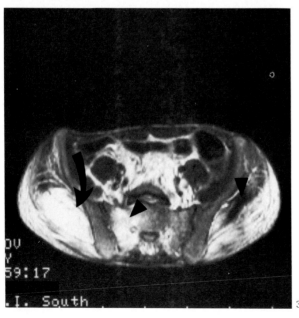

Figure 1 demonstrates a focal, fairly well-defined area of high signal with a mass effect (open arrow). Figure 2 is a slightly different cut; the curved arrow points to the abscess collection. An arrowhead points to the normal gluteal muscle on the left side. Another arrowhead points to the slight increase in the signal of the sacrum at the sacroiliac joint, suggesting that the infection may also be involving the sacral bone.

Figure 3 is a T2-weighted image again demonstrating the gluteal mass (curved arrow). Contrast this to the gluteal muscle on the left side, which is normal (arrowhead).

Another arrowhead points to the increased signal in the sacrum, suggesting that the abscess may also have involved the sacrum on the right side.

By signal characteristics alone, excluding a malignant process in this area would be difficult. However, the clinical history of pain, fairly accelerated growth, and clinical sepsis, in addition to the patient's young age and the absence of any history or suspicion of malignancy, aid in the diagnosis of large soft tissue abscess. MRI is useful in delineating the collection and its relationship to the soft tissue structures. Excellent bone detail is available. The cortex still appears intact, and despite the relative lack of involvement of the iliac bone on the right, there is a suspicion that the infection has spread and is probably involving the right sacral bone. The exact path of this infection is not clear. However, Figure 4a demonstrates that the infected material and fluid do extend beneath the sacroiliac joint (curved arrow). This may explain the apparent sparing of the iliac bone but involvement of the sacrum as the infection spreads back up into the right sacral region. MRI is uniquely suited to identify soft tissue structures such as this abscess. It is difficult to be specific without a clinical history, and a soft tissue malignancy would have to be considered without a clinical history of apparent sepsis. I think that there is a wealth of additional information because of the sensitivity to the change in bone mortar contents, as illustrated here. There would be no reason to suspect right sacral involvement until late bony destructive changes made it apparent on the basis of a plain film or CT investigation. The coronal views are also uniquely suited to augmenting this study in that they show the infectious material as it sweeps under the sacroiliac joint to involve the right sacrum (curved arrow, Figure 4b). Contrast this to the appearance on the left side (open arrow).

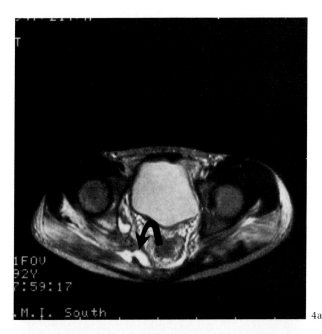

4a

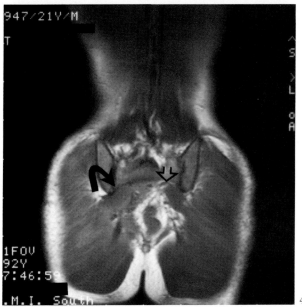

4b

8.5 PELVIC INFLAMMATORY MASS

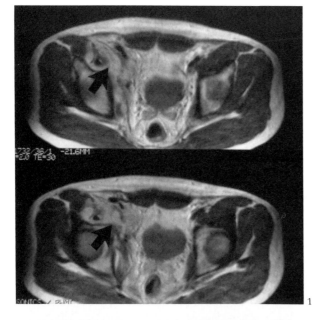

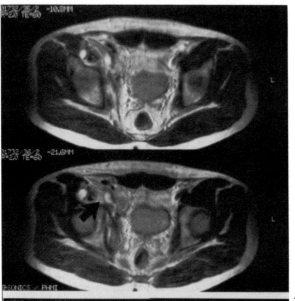

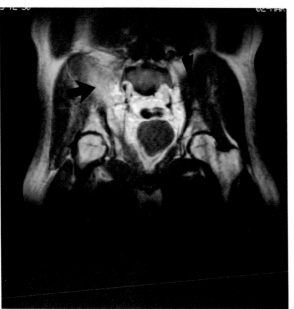

Figure 1 demonstrates a large amount of fluid and a non-specific collection surrounding the femoral artery and vein (large arrow). Note that the abnormal area is defined by MRI but lacks a definite mass and has a fairly homogeneous signal as it surrounds the psoas muscle and vessels.

Figure 2 is a T2-weighted image through these same cuts illustrating a slight increase in a portion of the abscess collection. The vessels and intact muscles can be identified as they pass through this inflammatory mass.

Figure 3 (short-stemmed arrow) is the coronal representation of this mass as it extends along the pelvis anterior to the iliac bone. Contrast this to the normal appearance of the iliopsoas muscle on the left (long-stemmed arrow).

This mass was originally interpreted by the radiologist as representing a sarcoma. However, it would be unusual for a mass of this size, particularly a sarcoma, to spare the adjacent bony cortex. Also, despite its large size, this mass appears to engulf or envelop the surrounding structures rather than to displace them, as would be suspected with most sarcomatous-type lesions. The entire extent of this abnormal mass was demonstrated nicely with MRI. Subsequent biopsy and treatment revealed this to be a large pelvic abscess and inflammatory fluid rather than sarcoma.

The signal characteristics of malignancy and abscess can overlap and be confusing; however, the physical properties of an abscess and a soft tissue tumor such as sarcoma help to differentiate them. As suspected, an inflammatory mass tends to engulf and surround rather than displace and form a discrete mass. Some infiltrative sarcomas that are more long-standing can infiltrate; however, because it was known clinically that the mass had appeared recently, abscess ultimately fit the diagnosis in retrospect.

MRI also augments this study by demonstrating the apparent lack of any bone infection complicating the presence of this pelvic mass.

8.6 DISCITIS OF THE L2–3 DISC SPACE

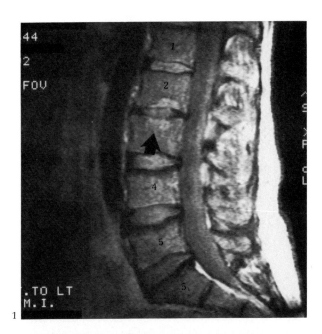

This is a very mild example of discitis. Figure 1 is a T1-weighted image through the abnormal disc. Note that there is loss of the normal cortical definition of the end plate, as well as alteration of signal within the bone marrow-containing spaces adjacent to the disc space. The disc signal intensity is slightly lower than that of the normal discs above and below it. Figure 2 demonstrates the T2-weighted appearance of this disc space. This very small amount of inflammation is difficult to differentiate from a degenerative disc. The helpful hint here is the loss of the normal cortical end plate definition, as well as the clinical findings, which are consistent with infection rather than degenerative changes. Figure 3 is an axial cut through the affected disc. It does not demonstrate any additional extension of the disease into the epidural space or the paraspinal region (large arrow).

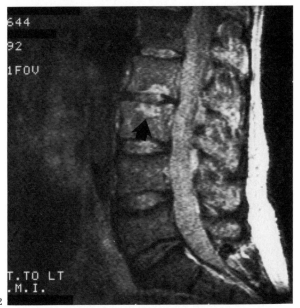

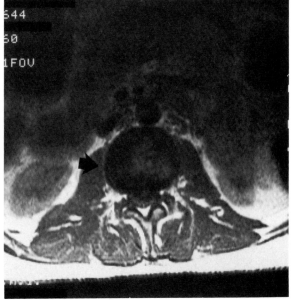

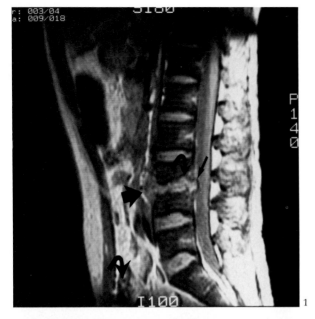

8.7 L4–5 DISCITIS

Figure 1 demonstrates the expanded appearance of a disc undergoing an inflammatory change, or discitis (large arrow). This is compared to the normal disc immediately below at L4–5 (small arrow). Note that the end plates have been disrupted and have altered detail, and there is expansion of the disc despite bulging both anteriorly and posteriorly (narrow arrow). Figure 2 is a T2-weighted image again demonstrating the infected L3–4 disc (large arrow). The epidural extension of material posteriorly is again identified. This can again be compared to the disc immediately below, which is entirely normal. The discitis and the initial infection can cause expansion. Following treatment and some decompression into the epidural space, the disc height is eventually lost. One key to a diagnosis of discitis is the erosion and destruction of the end plates, which can be identified in this case (curved arrow).

Figure 3 is an axial cut through the diseased disc. Note that the epidural fat demonstrated by the small arrows is compressed by the spread of the epidural mass (long-stemmed arrow). The thecal sac is slightly indented, but the overall sac does not appear to be invaded (arrow). The rootlets can be identified lying dependently in the inferior portion of the thecal sac with the patient supine.

The history is very helpful in making this diagnosis. However, a good rule of thumb is that infection seeks out relatively avascular cartilage, whereas malignancy tends to avoid this structure.

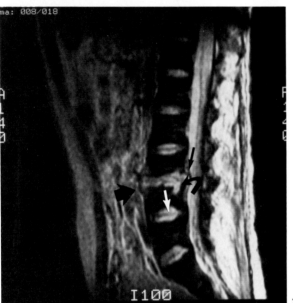

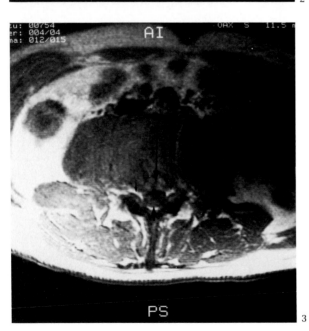

8.8 COMMINUTED FRACTURE OF THE HUMERUS WITH OSTEOMYELITIS

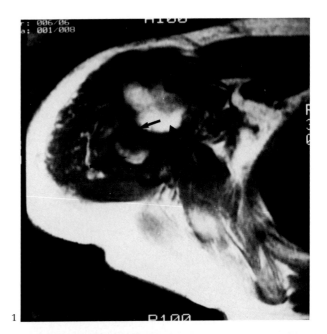

1

In this traumatized shoulder in a 35-year-old male (Figure 1), the rotated humeral head (large, short-stemmed arrow) is easily identified. The shaft (large, long-stemmed arrow) can also be seen. There is a large amount of fluid surrounding the fracture site. This is not atypical of an acute fracture representing hematoma and edema in the fracture region. The diagnosis of osteomyelitis superimposed on a fracture site requires a clinical history of fever and pain in excess of that expected for the fracture. In addition, this particular case demonstrates altered, decreased signal in the shaft distal to the fracture segment (large arrow, Figure 2a). Figure 2b demonstrates the humeral head rotated and dislocated from the shoulder joint (arrow). Figure 3 is a T2-weighted image again showing the effusion around the fracture site, which exhibits a high signal. There is no characteristic signal on a routine double-echo sequence to separate infected material from a mixture of hematoma and edema at the fracture site. In this T2-weighted image, the signal is suppressed in the bone marrow-containing humeral head (small white arrow).

The diagnosis of osteomyelitis in this case depended on clinical correlation. However, the extension of infection into the shaft and the amount of surrounding soft tissue and fluid in the fracture site were useful to the surgeons staging the infectious involvement and provided a useful method of follow-up for healing, as well as for assessing the response to antibiotics and/or any possible need to debride the infected region.

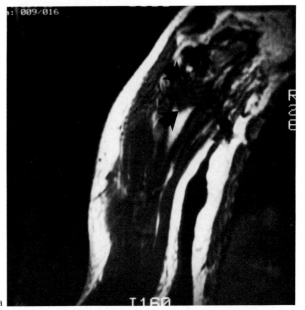

2a

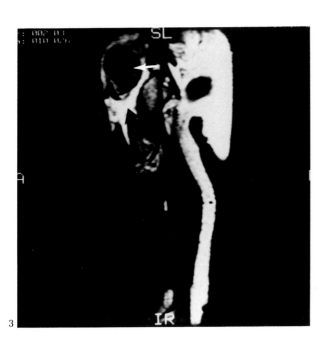

3

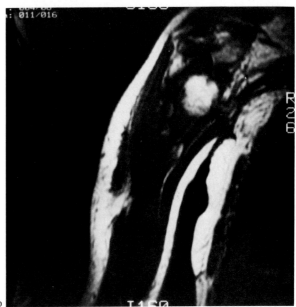

2b

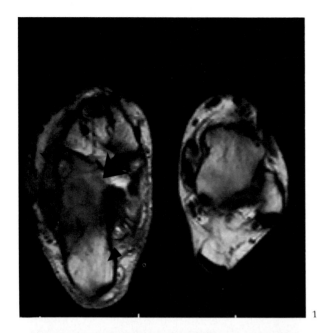

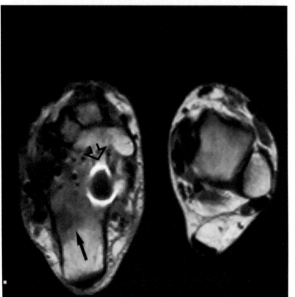

8.9 OSTEOMYELITIS OF THE CALCANEUS

This 45-year-old female demonstrates diffuse signal loss, as well as some cortical disruption of the anterior calcaneus (large arrow, Figure 1). This can be contrasted to the relatively uninvolved body of the calcaneus (arrowhead). Note that the infectious material extends into the subcutaneous tissue surrounding the bone and changes it from the normal high-signal subcutaneous fat to a more intermediate signal (open arrowhead). This surrounds the tendons in a diffuse, non-mass-producing fashion, unlike the extraosseous metastases shown earlier, which have a more definitive bulk and outline.

Figure 2 demonstrates the placement of a metal pin earlier for the purpose of stabilization. Despite the placement of this pin, note that there is relatively little degradation of the overall information available. On this slightly more inferior cut, the diffuse amount of bone edema extending into the calcaneus can also be identified, and the contrast is nicely illustrated (long-stemmed arrow).

Figure 3 is a coronal image demonstrating again the changes in the infected calcaneus versus a slightly more posterior cut through the uninvolved left calcaneus (arrows). Again, metal artifact can be seen where subtalar stabilization has been performed. Note that relatively little amount of information is lost despite the placement of metal pins.

Figure 4 is another cut through this same area, again contrasting the altered bone of the infected calcaneus. The subtalar joint has been narrowed secondary to attempts at stabilization as well as extension of infection. The large arrow points to the metal artifact. Contrast this to the normal appearance of the bone of the calcaneus on the left (small arrow). The curved arrow points to the infected calcaneus. The open arrow points to the effusion within the joint space.

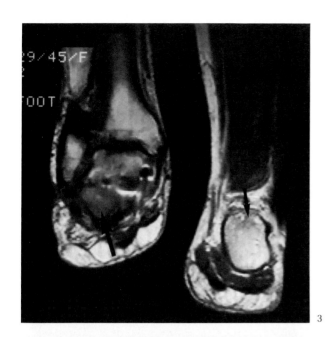

3

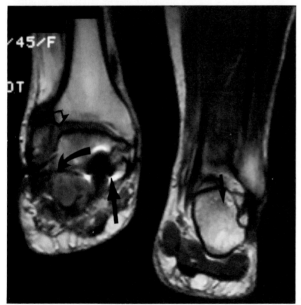

4

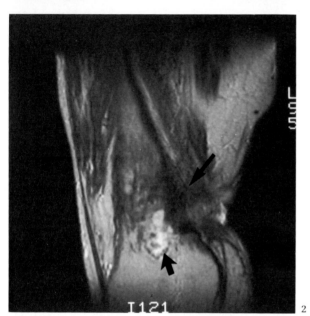

8.10 CHRONIC OSTEOMYELITIS OF THE FEMUR WITH A SINUS TRACT

Figure 1 is a coronal image demonstrating a cortical defect (large arrow). A sinus tract extending to the skin can be identified (long-stemmed arrow). The involucrum surrounded by inflammatory fluid can also be seen (short-stemmed arrow).

Figure 2 demonstrates these same features on a T2-weighted image. Note that some of the fluid and a portion of the involucrum now demonstrate increased signal. A large portion of the surrounding inflammatory change is chronic, and there has been squamous transformation of part of the tract.

Figure 3 is an axial image through the sinus tract. The cortical defect is identified (large-stemmed arrow). Air-fluid levels can be identified within the infected bone (small arrow). Large arrows demonstrate the infected fluid and outline its extent through the sinus tract to a defect in the skin representing the opening of the sinus tract externally.

Figure 4 demonstrates the appearance of this chronic osteomyelitis on a plain film. The arrow points to approximately the same position indicated on the coronal views.

MRI can easily identify the infected bone, involucrum, and sequestrum. In addition, the sinus tract can be identified, and the adjacent involvement of muscle or soft tissues can be well portrayed.

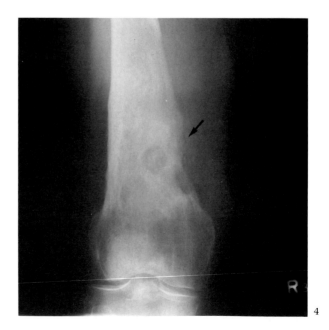

8.11 DISCITIS WITH EPIDURAL SPREAD

Figure 1 points to a herniated disc (long-stemmed arrow). Note the extension of the degenerative, inflammatory change into the midportion of the L3 vertebral body (solid arrow). Contrast this to the appearance of the end plate and disc at the normal level above (open arrow). Note also that the combination of herniated and infected, herniated material extends into the posterior canal, elevating the posterior longitudinal ligament (small arrow). Figure 2 demonstrates the high signal of the infected disc and infected, herniated fragments (long-stemmed arrow). The inflammatory changes and erosion into the vertebral body can be identified (solid arrow). Elevation of the posterior longitudinal ligament can be seen (small arrow).

On Figure 3, the axial images are also very instructive, demonstrating the confluence of the infected material as it spreads through the epidural space and along the paraspinal regions (short arrows). Note the axial cut of the extension of infection into the vertebral body (arrow). There is also right-sided spread into the paraspinal region (small arrow).

Figure 4 demonstrates the same changes in a slightly inferior cut.

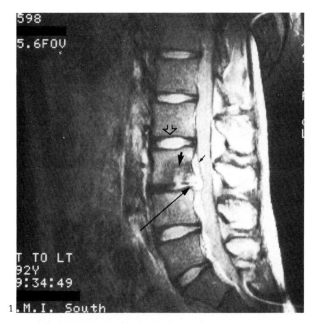

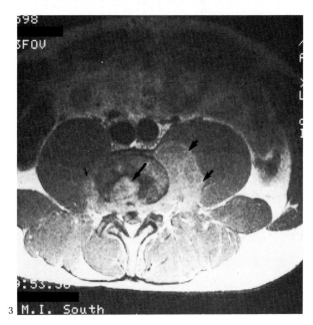

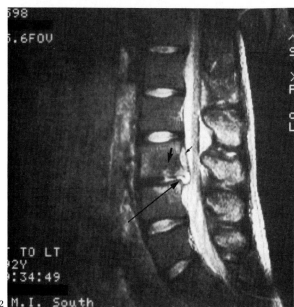

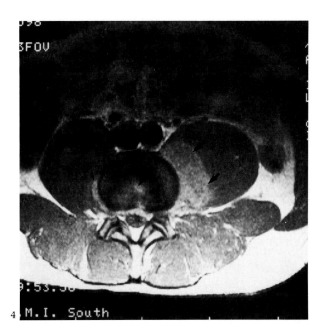

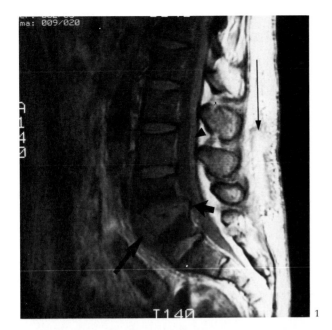

1

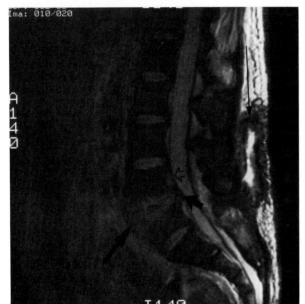

2

8.12 DISCITIS WITH EPIDURAL SPREAD

Figure 1 demonstrates expansion of the L4–5 disc and a large inflammatory mass (arrows). Note the extension posteriorly into the canal (short-stemmed, large arrow). The rootlets can be visualized (arrowhead). The tiny arrow points to one of the normal-appearing spinous processes. The long-stemmed arrow points to an area of prior surgical incision.

Figure 2 shows a signal that demonstrates a slight increase centrally on T2 weighting, but overall, the signal in the abnormal, expanded disc remains intermediate. Note that there is now high signal in the region of the incision (long-stemmed arrow). The posterior longitudinal ligament is slightly elevated above the herniated, infected material (open arrow).

Figure 3 demonstrates the diffuse loss of the normal disc (arrows). This also extends into and involves the left facet. The open arrow points to the thecal sac, and the high-signal epidural fat posterior to the thecal sac is normal.

Figure 4 is a more extreme left parasagittal cut. The epidural spread of material is demonstrated by the intermediate-signal mass (curved arrows). Note that the spread not only involves the L4–5 canal but also extends into the left neuroforaminal canal at the L5–S1 level. Contrast this to the high signal of the normal fat that exits through an upper neuroforaminal canal (open arrow).

Discitis is represented by altered signal, as well as by destruction of the end plate; the center of the process arises from the cartilage. The spread into the epidural space is sheet-like rather than a mass extension and is characteristic of discitis. Metastasis involves bone, and avoids or may totally envelope the cartilaginous disc.

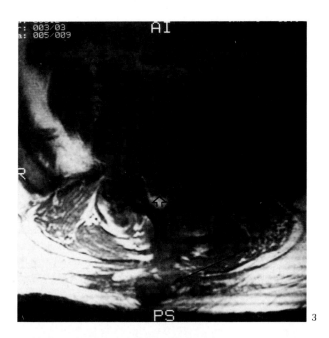

3

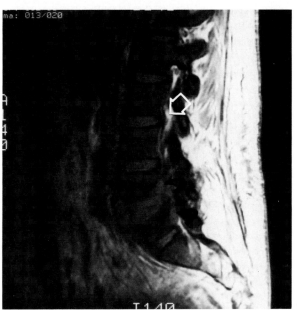

4

251

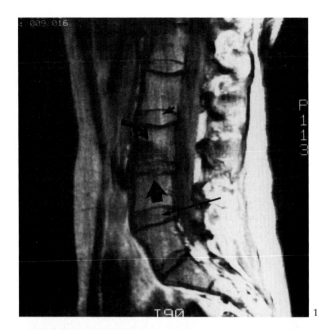

1

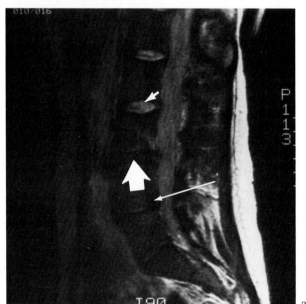

2

8.13 DISCITIS TO THE LUMBOSACRAL SPINE

This 30-year-old female presented with clinical findings of infection. Figure 1 is a T1- or proton density-weighted image of the lumbar spine. Figure 2 is a T2-weighted image. The small arrow demonstrates the appearance of the normal disc above the affected L3–4 level (large arrow). There is degenerative change in contrast to the infection and the normal disc (long-stemmed arrow) at the L4–5 level. Note that centrally there is a slight increase in signal on the T1-weighted and T2-weighted images (large arrows).

I have found that very early discitis is difficult to differentiate from a severely degenerative disc. Many of the findings, such as alteration of the end plate, narrowing of the disc, and alteration of signal within the disc, can overlap. Again, as mentioned in previous cases, it is essential that the clinical history and physical findings help to clarify the diagnosis. This particular case also demonstrates more end plate reaction than degeneration within the disc, which I would suggest is compatible with degenerative changes alone. Note that at L3 the decrease in signal extends up to the midbody (curved arrow).

8.14 TALAR OSTEOMYELITIS

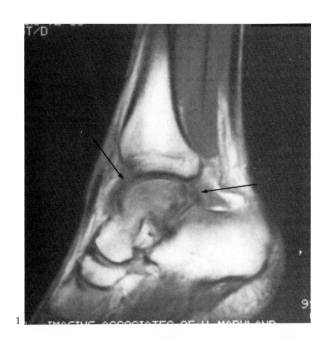

Figure 1 demonstrates diffuse signal loss and some cortical demineralization (long-stemmed arrows) of the talar bone. Figure 2a is a coronal cut through the normal left talar bone and the affected right talar bone. Note the loss of signal and some thinning of the cortices of the affected talus (long-stemmed arrow) in contrast to the normal talus (short arrow). Figure 2b also demonstrates the presence of joint effusion in the subtalar region (curved arrow) of the abnormal talus. Instead of the normal suppression of the bone marrow signal there is a diffuse increase in signal (long-stemmed arrow). Contrast this to the normal talus on the left (short-stemmed arrow). Figure 3 is an axial cut through the talus demonstrating again the diffuse signal loss, as well as the diffuse signal change representing edema and a soft tissue reaction to the infection surrounding the talus (short-stemmed arrows).

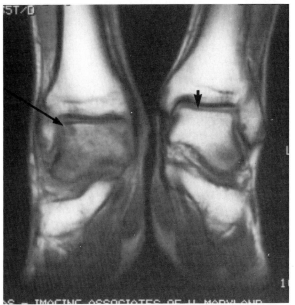

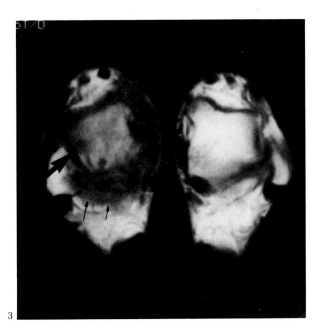

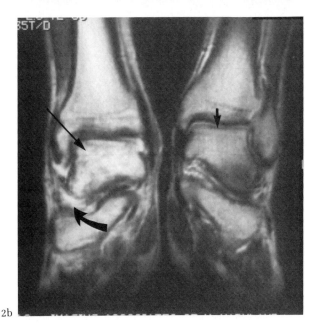

253

8.15 ABSCESS POSTERIOR IN THE ILIACUS MUSCLE

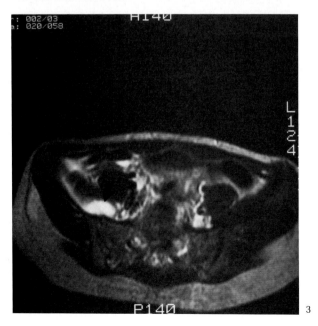

This is a 14-year-old female with pain upon movement of the psoas muscle. The studies done include a CT scan (Figure 1). A minimal low-density collection of fluid is suggested deep to the iliacus muscle (open arrowhead). The interface between this area and the posterior psoas is defined by the large arrow. This is fairly subtle and could be easily overlooked.

Figures 2 and 3 demonstrate a conspicuous increase in signal in the region of the sacroiliac joint consistent with a focal collection of fluid. Based on the signal characteristics, a chronic hematoma could not be differentiated from a collection of infected fluid at this level.

The MRI scan contrasts the abnormal tissue sharply with the subcutaneous fat and muscle, using the T1- and T2-weighted characteristics. Additional information, including the fact that the infected collection is larger than suggested on CT, was of use. The association and crossing of the sacroiliac joint was not well appreciated on the CT scan but is illustrated strongly on the MRI scan (see Figure 3).

8.16 OLD DISCITIS

There is marked loss of disc space and end plate irregularity at L2–3 (large arrows). Figure 1 is T1 weighted; Figure 2 is more T2 weighted. The absence of any increased signal or visualization of fluid within the disc suggests that the infection is now burnt out or low grade. There is no evidence of significant soft tissue mass or infected material. Alteration of the end plates in reaction to the infection is also identified. A minimal amount of osteophytic lipping is seen posterior to the disc space (curved arrow).

Figure 3 demonstrates the ostephytic lipping extending into the canal and slightly narrowing the canal space but not compressing the rootlets unduly (open arrow).

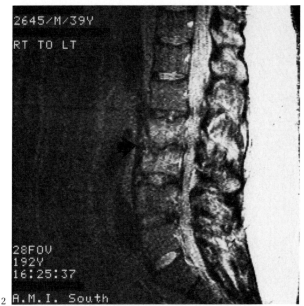

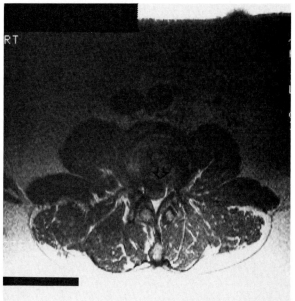

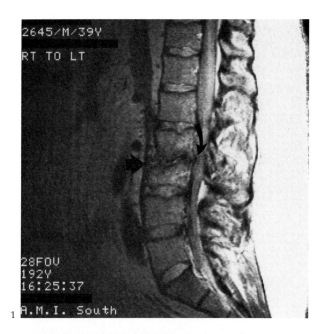

8.17 DECUBITUS ULCER

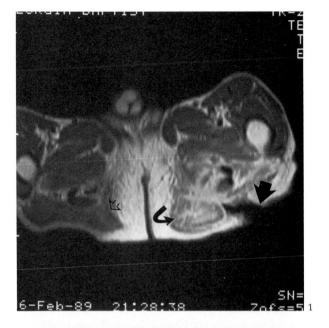

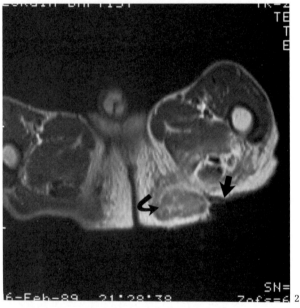

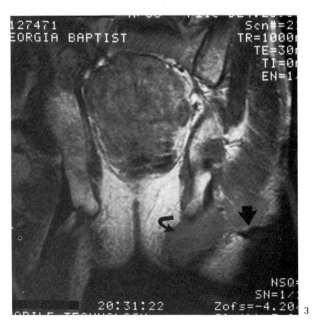

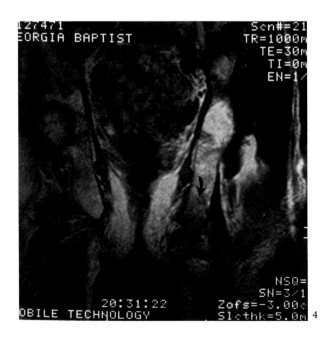

Figure 1 demonstrates decubitus breakdown and a large ulcer (large arrow). Deep and medial to the ulceration is a collection of fluid, which is not gluteal muscle (curved arrow). This is believed to represent an abscess collection. Contrast this to the normal appearance of the right gluteal musculature (open arrow). Figure 2 is a slightly different cut through the ulcer; the loss of the subcutaneous tissue identifies the defect. The mass is identified by the curved arrow. Figure 3 is a coronal image demonstrating the abscess in the coronal plane deep to the ischial tuberosity (curved arrow). The ulceration and skin defect can again be visualized (large arrow).

Figure 4 demonstrates loss of cortex in the ischial tuberosity, as well as altered signal in the bone, which is suggestive of extension of infection into the bone consistent with osteomyelitis (arrow). The cortical defect is seen in the inferior portion as the bone abuts the infectious collection of material (open arrow).

8.18 THORACIC DISCITIS WITH OSTEOMYELITIS AND EPIDURAL SPREAD

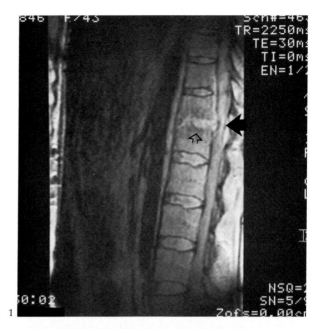

Figure 1 demonstrates a slightly expanded and altered signal with alteration of the end plate consistent with discitis (open arrow). This occurs in the lower thoracic region. Note that the epidural spread of material extends into the canal, causing canal narrowing (large arrow). Figure 2 is a T2-weighted image demonstrating increased signal in the infected disc. This indicates destruction of the intrameniscal septum. Alteration of the end plate and the epidural spread posteriorly, with canal compression, are again identified (large arrow). Figure 3a is a coronal image demonstrating the destruction of the disc and the paraspinal spread of material (arrows). Figure 3b, an axial cut, again demonstrates the spread of paravertebral soft tissue (curved arrow). Note the destructive changes in the left lateral disc space; cortical destruction can also be identified (solid arrow). Contrast this to the preserved cortex on the right (open arrow).

One further observation regarding the differentiation between osteomyelitis and metastasis is that osteomyelitis tends to extend in a symmetric fashion, as would any fluid. Note that on Figure 3b there is nonspecific fluid encasing the posterior aspect of the aorta, as well as surrounding and extending on both sides of the vertebral disc space. Metastatic disease, despite its severity, usually lacks a fairly symmetric appearance. Other differences, such as changes beginning in the disc space instead of bone, help to differentiate infection, which favors disc space origin, from metastasis, which favors bone origin and avoids cartilage or avascular structures.

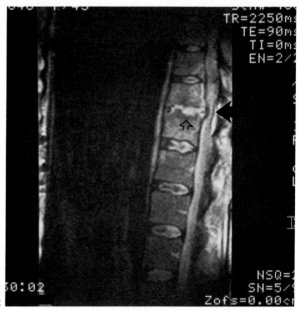

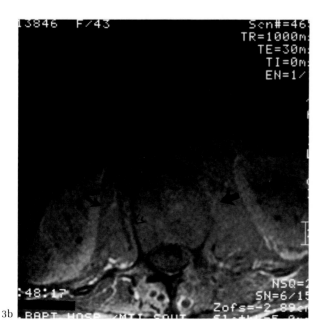

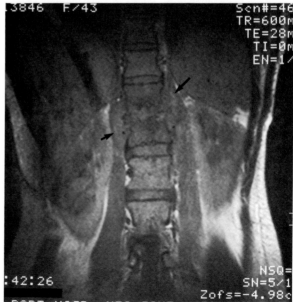

8.19 OSTEOMYELITIS OF THE CALCANEUS WITH A PRESSURE ULCER AND A DIABETIC PATIENT

Figure 1 is a sagittal cut demonstrating pressure or decubitus ulceration (long-stemmed arrow). Note the inflammatory change in the subcutaneous tissues outlined by the small arrows. Contrast this to the noninvolved subcutaneous tissues adjacent to this change. The solid arrow points to the alteration of signal in the calcaneus, representing alteration of bone mortar secondary to edema and inflammatory hypercellularity. The interface between this and the more normal right signal of the noninfected marrow of the calcaneus is fairly well contrasted, although the margin is not sharp.

Figure 2 is a coronal image demonstrating the same loss of the normal high signal (arrows). Note that the ulceration can be identified, as well as breakdown of the actual epidermal layer (long-stemmed arrow). The inflammatory change and the subcutaneous tissues are nicely contrasted to the normal subcutaneous tissues in the more lateral and medial aspects of the foot.

Figure 3 is an axial cut through this infected talus. Note that the cortex posteriorly has been destroyed and lost. This can also be seen on Figures 1 and 2.

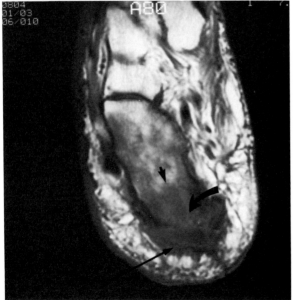

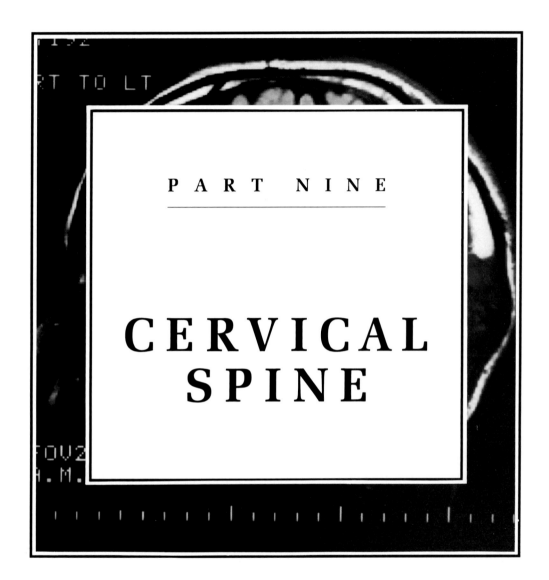

PART NINE

CERVICAL SPINE

9.1 SYRINX WITH HERNIATION

Figure 1 demonstrates multiple herniations (arrowheads). Immediately below the C6–7 herniation is a syrinx cavity (large arrow). This can be confirmed by the axial cut (Figure 2, curved arrow). Recent articles suggest that syrinx development can be related to external compression on the cervical cord, such as seen with herniations.

Figure 3 demonstrates, on the same patient, an incidental high-signal structure arising in the posterior fossa (large-stemmed arrow). It appears to be related to or arising from the posterior aspect of the tectal plate (large arrow). High signal usually reflects increased fatty content. This is most likely an incidental lipoma or possibly a dermoid. The lack of hydrocephalus in this patient suggests that this is a benign incidental lesion.

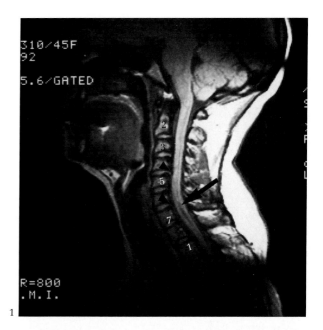

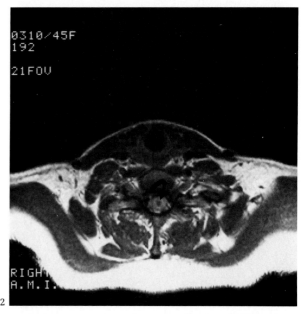

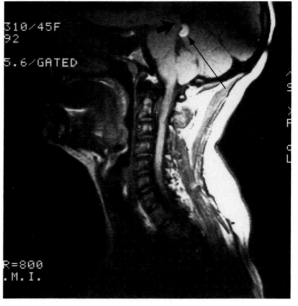

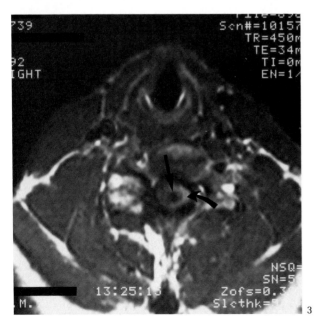

9.2 OLD CERVICAL TRAUMA WITH FUSION AND DEVELOPMENT OF CYSTIC MYELOMALACIA

Figure 1 demonstrates a fusion at the C6–7 level secondary to old trauma (open arrowhead). The large arrow points to the largely transected cord at the C6 level. Note that some elements of intact neural tissues span the area of damage (small arrows).

Figure 2 is an axial cut above the level of maximal injury demonstrating a syrinx-type cavity that has extended into the right half of the cord (large arrow).

Figure 3, a slightly lower cut, demonstrates the enlarging amount of cystic damage in the cord (large arrow). The preserved cord to the left of the midline is identified by the curved arrow. The lower axial cuts demonstrate even more loss of normal tissue and the presence of syrinx, as well as cystic end-stage cord myelomalacia.

9.3 CHIARI I MALFORMATION WITH EXTENSIVE SYRINX

Figure 1, a scout sagittal cut, demonstrates a congenitally low cerebellar tonsil (open arrow). This is not associated in this patient with evidence of a myelomeningocele and is consistent with a Chiari I malformation. These malformations are generally detected in young adults, and their presentation can be quite confusing. A common associated finding is a syrinx. In this case, an extensive syrinx (large arrows) extends from the C2–3 level to the T9 level.

Figure 2 is a surface coil sagittal cut through the same area. Again note the low position of the cerebellar tonsil reaching to the level of the posterior bony arch of C1 (open arrow). The foramen magnum is identified by the long-stemmed arrow. The large arrow points to the superior aspect of the syrinx, and the arrowheads demonstrate bands or septations across the syrinx cavity that probably represent disrupted neural connections between the separated portions of the cervical cord.

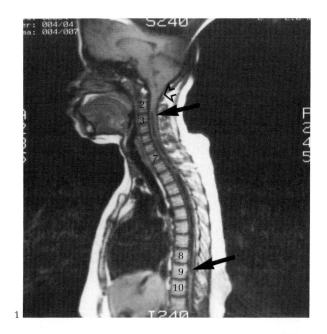

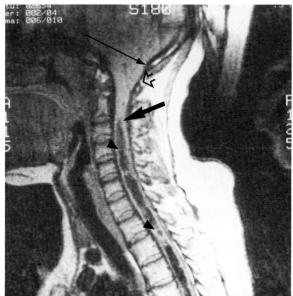

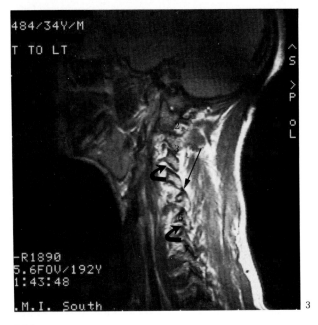

9.4 POSTTRAUMATIC HERNIATION WITH PERCHED FACET

Figure 1 demonstrates large herniations at the C4–5 and C5–6 levels. Note that the C5–6 level maintains a low degenerative appearance, whereas the C4–5 level is increased in signal throughout, and there is evidence of caudal extension of the disc herniation. The T2-weighted image on Figure 2 demonstrates the diffuse increase in signal of this defect, suggesting that there is hemorrhage and that this herniation is acute. The open arrow demonstrates hematoma, which is tracked along the prevertebral soft tissues. Note that the C5–6 disc herniation maintains a low signal and is consistent with having been present prior to the trauma (large arrows). In this patient, there is an excellent example of perched facets. Note that the C4 facet is perched atop the C5 facet (Figure 3, long-stemmed arrow), which is consistent with severe flexion injury and disruption of the facet capsule at this level. The normal alignment of the C2–3 and C3–4 levels above can be nicely identified, as can the normal alignment of C6–7 and C7 on T1 below (curved arrows).

9.5 OS ODENTUM WITH SUBLUXATION AND HYPERTROPHY OF THE TRANSVERSE LIGAMENT AND UNDERLYING CORD COMPRESSION

Figure 1 demonstrates the separation of the dens from the base of the C2 vertebral body. The separated dens is now referred to as an *os odentum*. The fibrous cleft between the os and the body of C2 can be identified on Figure 1 (small arrow). The os odentum is designated by the curved arrow.

More important is the hypertrophic changes within the transverse ligament, which cause marked underlying cord compression at the C2 level (large arrow).

Figure 2 (small arrow) demonstrates the fibrous area now represented by increased signal. The cord compression is again identified (large arrow). Importantly, an area superior to the maximal area of compression shows increased signal and suggests alteration of water content within the cord, reflecting edema and possibly myelomalacia (open arrow).

Figure 3 is an axial cut through the level of compression. The curved arrow points to the hypertrophied transverse ligament. Also note the presence of the thinned, compressed cervical cord (open arrow).

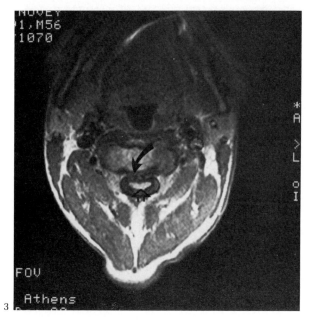

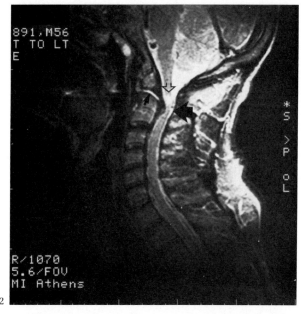

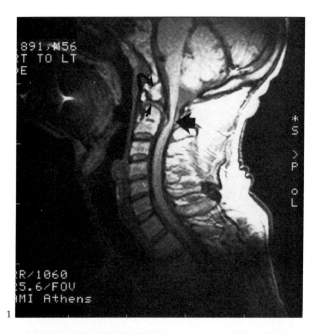

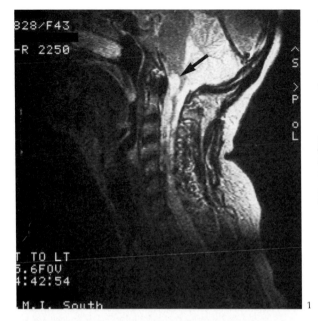

9.6 MULTIPLE SCLEROSIS (MS) IN THE MEDULLARY AND UPPER CERVICAL CORD REGION

Figure 1 demonstrates a large plaque-like area of signal involving the medullary and upper cervical regions. Figures 2 and 3 (large arrows) demonstrate the involvement of the left half of the medullary brain stem and the upper cervical cord on T1 or proton density weighting on Figure 2 and T2-weighting on Figure 3.

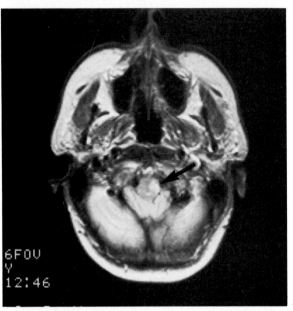

9.7 MS PLAQUE IN THE CERVICAL REGION

Figure 1 demonstrates a plaque represented by a flame-shaped, high signal at the C2–3 level within the cord. Note that this requires routine double-echo images and is invisible on the T1-weighted image (Figure 2, large arrow).

It is important to recognize that MS can involve the cervical or thoracic cord. This is usually not associated with a normal cranial study, but the head is spared in rare cases, and a focal isolated plaque can be present in the cord. The presentation of MS is protean. The high level of detection available with MRI helps to prevent the clinical investigator from overlooking this possibility.

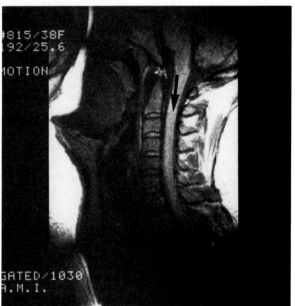

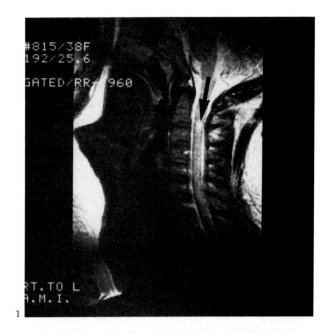

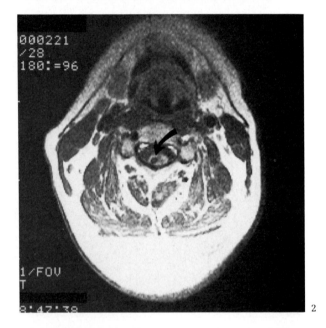

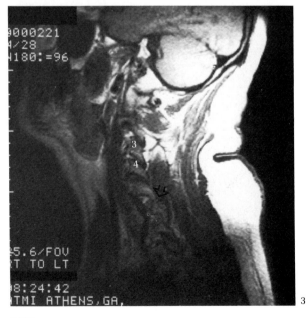

9.8 OLD TRAUMA WITH FUSION AND SYRINX WITH OLD LOCKED JUMP FACET

Figure 1 (large arrow) demonstrates anterior vertebral body fusion secondary to correction of cervical trauma in the past. The underlying cord has generated a large syrinx cavity (small arrows). This extends up to the foramen magnum and into the thoracic region.

Figure 2 demonstrates the syrinx in an axial cut through the upper cervical spine.

Figure 3 demonstrates the abnormal alignment of the C5 and C6 facets. The C5 facet has ridden slightly past the C6 facet and is now in a locked position. This problem was not reduced with prior surgery.

The sequelae of trauma to the cord can be nicely demonstrated by MRI. The evolvement of syrinxes and cystic encephalomalacia and the progression of the cyst may explain the late onset of neurological difficulties in the traumatized cord.

The alignment of the vertebral bodies following reduction or internal fixation can also be identified. Equally valuable is the demonstration of the facets and their alignment in the traumatized cervical vertebral column.

9.9 TRAUMATIC HERNIATION IN THE CERVICAL SPINE

Figure 1 demonstrates another flexion injury, with C5 anterior to C6. Traumatic herniation of material is identified, with marked cord compression (curved arrow). Figure 2 demonstrates the flexed and abnormally subluxed position of the C5 facet on C6, creating a perched appearance.

The apparent second head is a wraparound artifact secondary to technical factors from the choice of field of view. It represents the anterior portion of the image not included in the true image (curved arrows).

This case is through the courtesy of Dr. Walter Bednarz of Williamsport Magnetic Imaging.

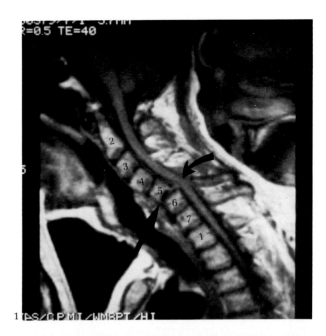

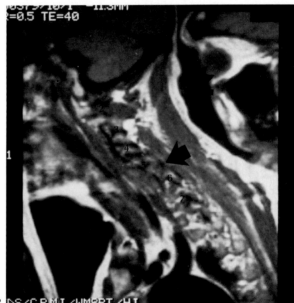

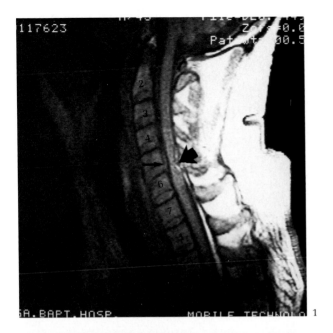

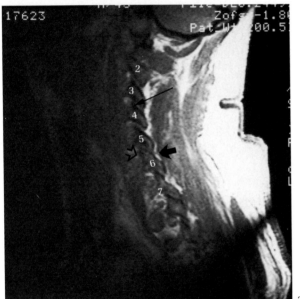

9.10 TRAUMATIC HERNIATION SECONDARY TO FLEXION INJURY WITH UNDERLYING CORD DAMAGE AND FACET FRACTURE

Figure 1 demonstrates marked wasting secondary to cord damage following flexion injury at the C5–6 level. Traumatically herniated disc can also be identified (small arrow).

Figure 2 demonstrates the perched appearance of the C5 facet on the C6 facet (large arrow). In addition, a small fragment from the C6 facet is identified (open arrow). Compare this with the normal alignment of the C3 and C4 and C4 on C5 facets, and note the intact appearance of the facet anteriorly at C4 (long-stemmed arrow).

I would like to see MRI used for front-line assessment of cervical cord trauma. It has the capability of showing the alignment of the vertebral bodies. It can clearly define facet injuries and their alignment and, most importantly, can show the condition of the cervical cord, which is the most crucial assessment necessary. Most trauma patients we have imaged have not required extensive ventilator assistance and could be monitored safely using the existing telemetry devices. However, some ventilators are resistant to magnetic fields. Several leading academic institutions are moving to incorporate MRI as a front-line imaging modality in the field of trauma medicine.

9.11 C2–3 DISC HERNIATION

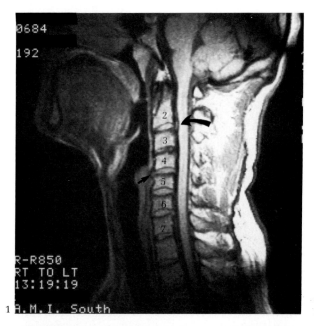

The upper cervical levels are frequently overlooked with the standard CT techniques employed today. However, MRI routinely includes the area from the foramen magnum to about the second thoracic vertebral body, and we have encountered a large number of herniations in the upper cervical region. Figure 1 is a nice example of a herniation at the C2–3 level (curved arrow). Figure 2 is a T2-weighted image confirming the presence of the herniation (curved arrow).

Figure 3 is an axial cut through the herniation (curved arrow). Note that the cord is also indented at this level (open arrow) and that the presence of herniations in the upper cord can significantly impinge upon the cord.

Figure 2 also demonstrates that the degenerative loss of signal can be verified at the C3–4 through C6–7 levels. Note the anterior osteophyte at the C4–5 level (small arrow).

Now go back to Figure 1. Did you notice the herniation at C6–7?

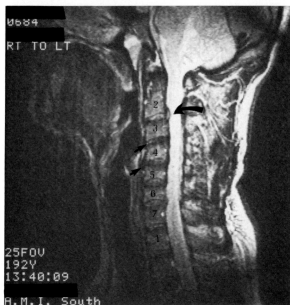

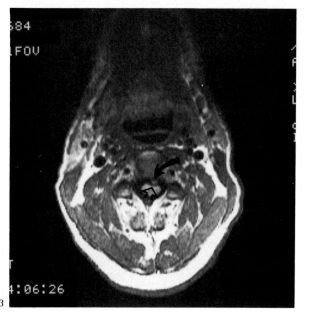

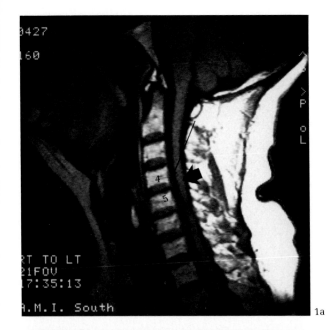

1a

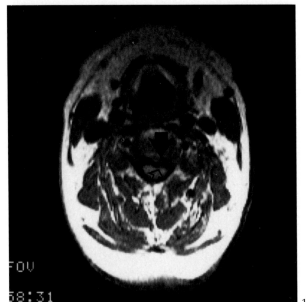

1b

9.12 THREE LARGE, CONTIGUOUS EXTRADURAL DEFECTS IN THE CERVICAL SPINE INVOLVING C4–5, C5–6, AND C6–7

Figure 1a demonstrates a large, soft tissue-type herniation at C5–6. The posterior aspects of the vertebral bodies can be identified within this mass, and no osteophyte is suggested (long-stemmed arrow). Figure 1b is an axial cut demonstrating the herniation (large arrow) and the flattening of the cord secondary to this defect (open arrow).

Figure 2a demonstrates a slightly larger defect at the C5–6 level. Note that the end plates are not as well visualized and that the presence of osteophyte and bone in the defect is suggested (small arrows).

Figure 2b demonstrates the defect (large arrow). Even more marked cord compression is evident on the axial and sagittal scans at this level (open arrow).

The C6–7 level demonstrates a similar large defect representing herniation. Figure 3a (long-stemmed arrows) demonstrates a significant osteophyte arising from the posterior aspect of the C7 superior end plate that contributes to this defect. Note that the cortical low density from C7 can be followed contiguously along this defect, helping to ensure at diagnosis that at least a portion of this defect is secondary to osteophytic development.

Figure 2b (open arrow) again demonstrates cord compression at the C6–7 level.

When such contiguous, large defects are present in the cervical spine, one should also include or assess for the possibility of calcification of the posterior longitudinal ligament. This is seen in Forestier's disease. This calcification can assume large, mass-like shapes and cause significant compression of the cord. Inspection of these three vertebral disc spaces demonstrates communication of the disc with the defect and identifies the osteophyte. It also helps to explain the defects as the combination of herniation and osteophyte at C5–6 and C6–7 and predominantly as herniation at the C4–5 level.

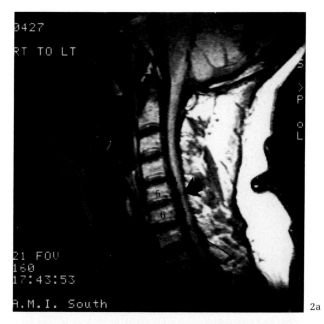

2a

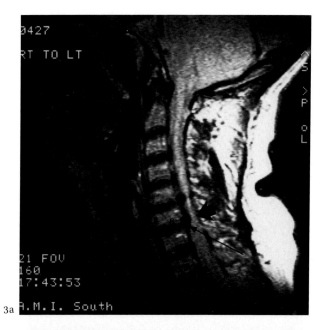

3a

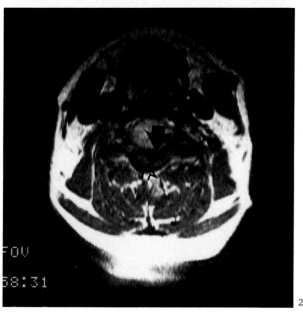

2b

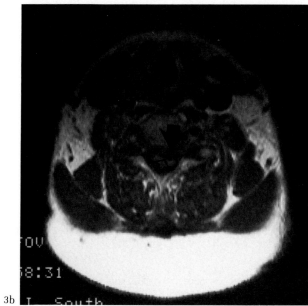

3b

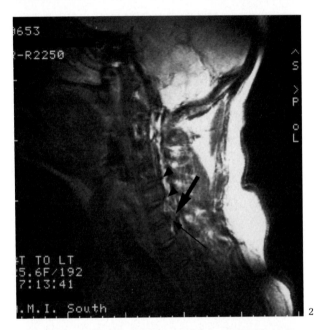

9.13 LARGE RIGHT C6–7 DISC HERNIATION

Figure 1 is an axial image demonstrating nicely the large disc herniation at the C6–7 level (large arrow). Note that there is also a mass effect upon the cord (open arrow). Incidental note is made of how well the jugular and carotid arteries can be visualized on these axial images and their lumens assessed. There is much current interest among neuroradiologists in evaluating arteriosclerosis with MRI as a screening modality (curved arrows).

Figure 2, a T1- or proton density-weighted image, demonstrates the defect in the extreme right parasagittal cut (large arrow). Note the absence of a similar defect at the two levels immediately above, which is nicely contrasted by the high signal of the epidural fat (arrowheads).

The advantage of double-echo imaging is that the sagittal image on the T1-weighted image can be confirmed with the myelographic appearance of the T2-weighted image (Figure 3, large arrow).

Figure 2 (long-stemmed arrow) also demonstrates the lipped appearance of the vertebral end plates and suggests an osteophytic component to the extradural defect.

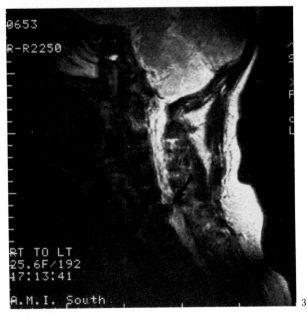

274

9.14 C5–6 DISC HERNIATION WITH MILD CORD FLATTENING

Figure 1 demonstrates a disc herniation at C5–6. Note that the material is similar in intensity to the material remaining between the C5 and C6 vertebral bodies. Note also that the material outlines the posterior aspect of the vertebral bodies and that little or no suggestion of osteophytic lipping is present (large-stemmed arrows point to the vertebral body outlines at the level of the defect).

Figure 2 demonstrates that disc herniations, like degenerating discs, can be increased rather than decreased in signal. This also demonstrates the mass effect upon the cord (large arrow). In this case, the presence of increased signal above and below the defect (long-stemmed arrows) reflects distention of the cervical epidural veins. Care must be taken not to miss a free fragment. In the recent literature, free fragments have also been demonstrated to be revascularized to explain the increased signal.

Figure 3 is an axial cut through the C5–6 disc space. The defect is identified nicely by the large arrow. The open arrow points to the slight indentation or compression of the cord (open arrow). The rootlets can also be identified within the canal (small arrow) and exiting past the disc herniation and posterior to the vertebral body (curved arrow). The long-stemmed arrow points to the vertebral artery.

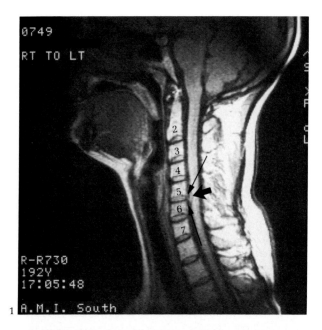

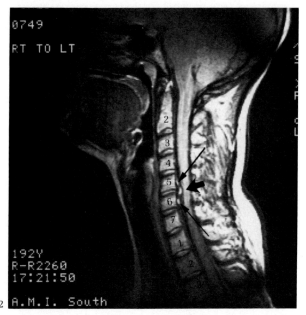

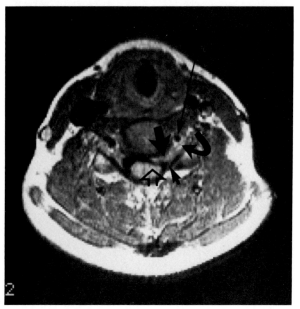

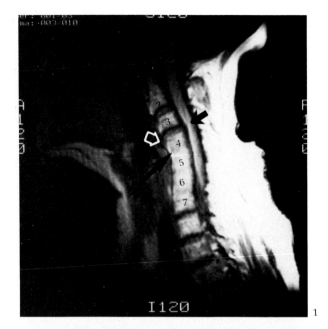

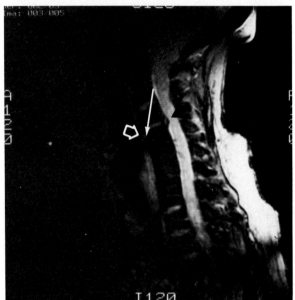

9.15 HERNIATION OCCURRING ABOVE A THREE-LEVEL FUSION

Figure 1 demonstrates the appearance of fusions at the C4–5, C5–6, and C6–7 levels (large arrow). Note that a defect is suggested at the C3–4 level; the cord is indented at this level. This is a proton density image. There has been slight motion degradation of the image.

Figure 2 is a gradient echo sagittal view accentuating the T2 factors and creating a myelographic effect. The defect is more clearly illustrated on this cut (large arrow). The herniation is nicely illustrated, and its slight mass effect upon the cord can also be appreciated. Note that the fusion levels appear intact, and no extradural defects at these levels are suggested. The long-stemmed white arrow points to an anterior herniation of the disc at the C3–4 level. This can be useful in verifying a suspected posterior herniation, since annular degeneration is not a focal disease of the posterior annulus alone, but rather a diffuse disease. In addition, anterior herniations, although usually clinically incidental, can be seen with a degenerative disc, indicating secondarily that herniation suspected posteriorly is probably real. This is also a demonstration of a large anterior osteophyte at the C3–4 level. Note that the signal on Figures 1 and 2 of this large anterior osteophytic lip extending from C3 is similar to that of the vertebral body bone (open arrows).

9.16 C3–4 AND C4–5 SPONDYLOTIC BARS

Figure 1 demonstrates a bulging annulus at the C3–4 and C4–5 levels (large arrows). In addition, some of the decreased signal includes osteophyte. The combination of an osteophytic spur and a bulging annulus is referred to collectively as a *bar* or a *spondylotic bar*. The presence of a bar is more common than a simple herniation of material in the cervical region. In either case, the presence of an extradural defect is not well tolerated in the cervical canal. MRI allows definition of the levels of involvement, as well as the amount of cord compression or root deviation associated with these defects.

Figure 2 demonstrates left-sided extension of the bar into the left central and neuroforaminal canals at these levels (large arrows). Figure 3 is a T2-weighted image that again verifies and confirms the presence of these defects as they extend into the canal. This image gives information on the degenerative nature of the disc at C3–4 and C4–5. Note that, in addition to these abnormalities, there is loss of disc signal at the C2–3 and C5–6 levels, revealing degeneration but not demonstrating any extradural defect at these levels. More normal signal is resumed at the C6–7 and C7–T1 levels (long-stemmed arrows point to the degenerative disc at C2–3 and C5–6).

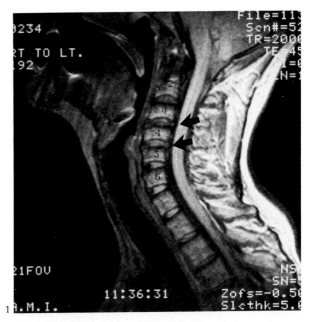

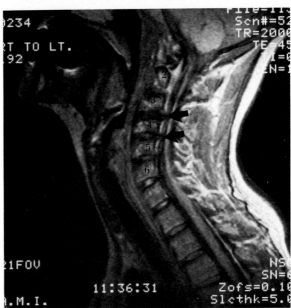

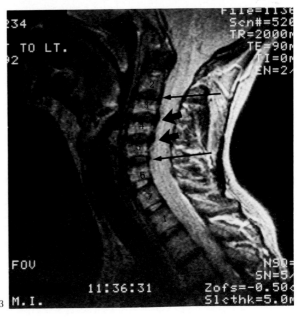

9.17 C6–7 DISC HERNIATION

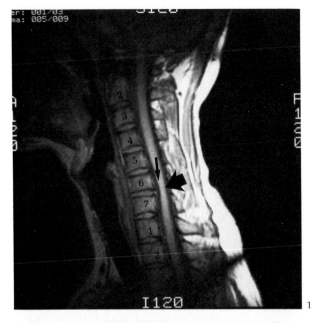

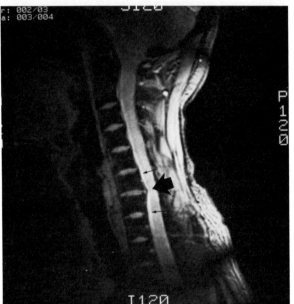

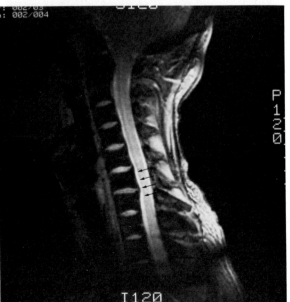

This is a 22-year-old male. Figure 1 demonstrates the loss of cervical lordosis with a degenerative or herniated disc. The vertebral bodies align in a fairly vertical fashion rather than in a soft cervical lordotic curve. The extradural defect can be identified at the C6–7 level (large arrow). The cord is compressed (small arrow).

Figure 2, using gradient echo technique, provides a T2-weighted image with a myelographic effect in a shorter period of time. Note that the herniated disc is shown to even better effect (large arrow). At initial inspection, the cord appears to have been lost in the enhanced cerebrospinal fluid (CSF). However, Figures 2a and 2b (small arrows) demonstrate the separation of the cord from the CSF interface (small arrows).

Figure 3a, an axial study, again using gradient echo technique, allows visualization of the herniated disc (large arrow) and the mass effect upon the cord (small arrow). This rivals the myelographically enhanced CT scan for detection of herniations. However, in combination with the sagittal images, MRI should clearly be the modality of choice in detecting disc herniation in the vertebral column.

Figure 3b demonstrates nicely the enhancement of the anterior and posterior nerve roots as they exit through the right neuroforaminal canal (curved arrow).

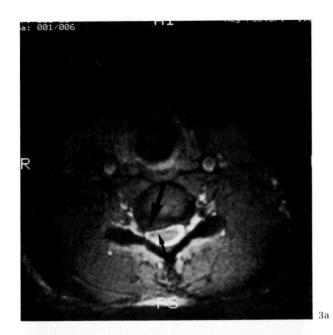

3a

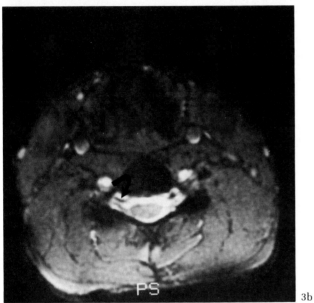

3b

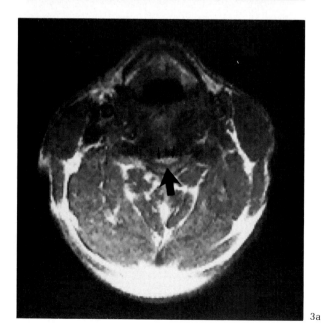

9.18 WASHERBOARD SPINE WITH CORD COMPRESSION

Figure 1 demonstrates large defects at the C4–5 and C5–6 levels. A similar defect is present at C3–4. More importantly, the cord, which is visualized as the area of intermediate high signal running within the canal, is markedly deformed. The cord can be differentiated from CSF, which is identifiable at C2 and C7 (small arrows). In addition, a focus of increased signal from C3–4 through C4–5 within the cord suggests edema and underlying myelomalacia.

Figure 2, a T2-weighted image, further verifies the severe narrowing of the spinal canal at the C4–5 and C5–6 levels.

Figures 3a and 3b demonstrate the markedly atrophied and compressed appearance of the cord, which is designated anteriorly by the small arrows and posteriorly by the large arrows.

Acquired degenerative spondylosis of this severity with multiple levels of involvement has been referred to as a *washerboard spine*. This term can be used with varying degrees of underlying cord compression. The most significant finding is, of course, the degree of compression and cord deformity that is present. MRI is useful in identifying the extent of most severe canal stenosis. It can also identify the caudal and cranial extent of the stenosis. Additionally, its ability to visualize the underlying cord directly, and to verify and document the amount of damage, is very useful. The increased signal suggested on Figure 1 may alert the clinician to the presence of more acute cord damage. In this case, the cord has been chronically injured and has long been markedly atrophied, but the areas of increased signal may suggest a newer area of involvement and may indicate the changes in the patient's symptoms.

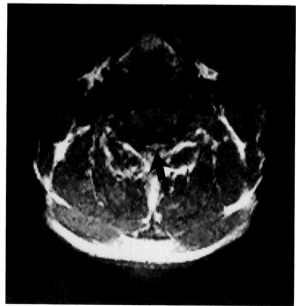

3a

3b

9.19 A C4–5 DISC HERNIATION WITH ASSOCIATED CORD COMPRESSION

Figure 1 demonstrates the disc herniation identified on the sagittal view (large arrow). The defect extends posterior to the vertebral bodies. There is also reversal of the upper portion of the normal cervical lordotic curvature. This reversal also involves the C3–4 level.

Figure 2 demonstrates the typical appearance of degenerative changes within the disc from C2–3 through C6–7. The T2-weighted images enhance the CSF and cause an MRI myelographic effect. The C4–5 defect can again be identified and confirmed.

The C5–6 level demonstrates a herniation as well a cleft through the normal low-signal annulus (large arrow). A defect is identified on Figure 2 in the myelographic T2-weighted images.

The identification of these herniations is most significant in that they can be related to their effect on the cord.

Marked compression is identified at the C4–5 level on the axial image (Figure 3). The large arrow demonstrates the large herniated defect in the right central canal. The small arrow shows the flattened, compressed cord.

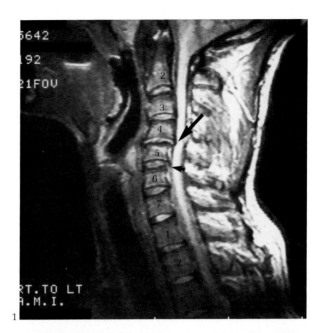

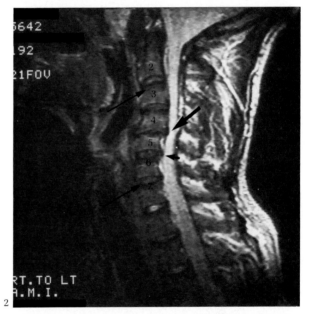

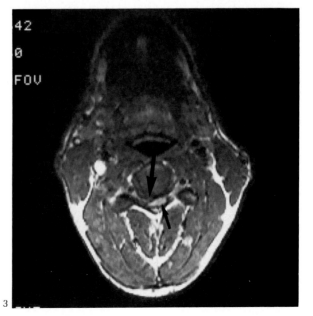

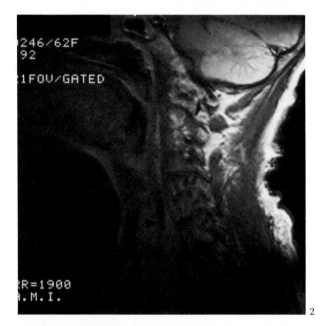

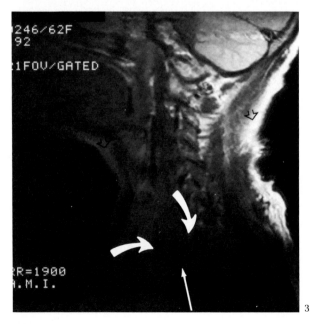

9.20 PARAVERTEBRAL MASS WITH SOME INVASION OF THE C5 VERTEBRAL BODY (LYMPHOMA)

Extreme parasagittal cuts can be very useful. On Figure 1, a predominantly extraosseous paraspinal mass can be observed (long-stemmed arrow). There is also direct invasion into the posterior aspect of the C5 vertebral body (arrowhead).

Figures 2 and 3, left-sided parasagittal cuts, outline the great vessels surrounded by diffuse tumor involvement, in this case proven to represent lymphoma. Note that the great vessel (arrowhead) is interspersed between the soft tissue neoplasm. On Figure 3, a vessel, probably a subclavian artery coursing through the mass, is identified as a rounded area of signal void (long-stemmed white arrow). The mass is an intermediate density structure that contrasts sharply to the other areas of soft tissue fat, which are higher in signal (open arrowheads).

This case illustrates the importance of photographing all of the images in an acquisition. The extreme parasagittal cuts, although excluding the central canal or the spine, can yield important information on the cause of radiculopathies. Note that the tumor, while invading the cervical vertebral body only minimally, is in a position to interfere with and entrap the exiting cervical nerves.

9.21 STATUS AFTER FUSION; RECURRENT OSTEOPHYTE EVIDENT WITH CORD COMPRESSION

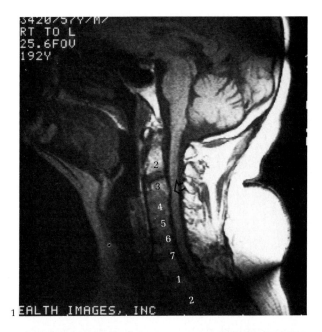

Figure 1 (open arrow) demonstrates an osteophyte rising from the now fused C3–4 disc level (open arrow). An indentation to the ventral aspect of the cord can be identified. Figure 2 is an axial image through this level that demonstrates the osteophyte extending into the left central and neuroforaminal canals (large arrow). The displacement of the cord is identified, and compression of the roots can be seen (small arrows). Figure 3 demonstrates a similar defect at the C5–6 level (open arrow). The axial image through this level on Figure 4 again demonstrates the large osteophytic structure extending into the left central canal (large arrow). Again, the compressed roots area can be seen (small arrow). In this example, the cord has also been slightly flattened, suggesting compression (open arrow).

Although the fusions at the C3–4, C4–5, and C5–6 levels appear solid, the osteophytic growth continued and the patient currently suffers from left-sided radiculopathy because of pressure upon the cord and roots secondary to bony osteophyte rather than disc material. In Figures 2 and 4, the signal is of intermediate intensity, with a well-defined cortical edge, and the signal of the defect is exactly that of the vertebral bodies. This allows a confident diagnosis that surgery will reveal bone rather than herniated material.

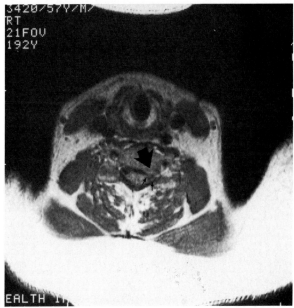

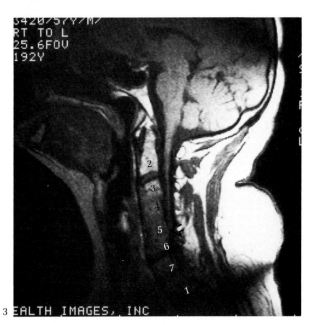

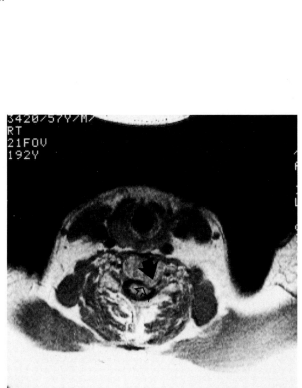

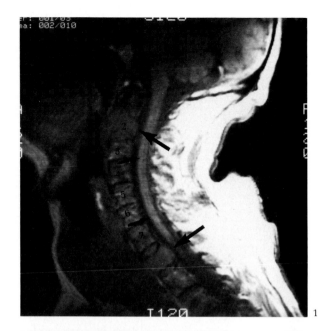

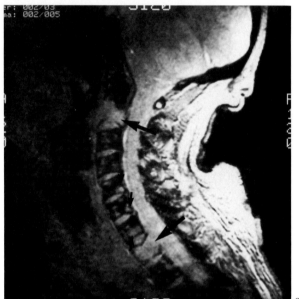

9.22 DIFFUSE CERVICAL BODY METASTASIS AT MULTIPLE LEVELS

Figure 1 demonstrates the blown-out appearance of a metastasis involving the body of C2 (large arrows). There is equally severe involvement of the T1 vertebral body (more inferior large arrow). Note that at T1 the body is bowing backward and touches, but has not yet compressed, the cord at this point of disease progression. Inspection of C3 through C7 also demonstrates the heterogeneous appearance of the cervical vertebral bodies. This heterogeneous appearance should suggest strongly that the metastasis has infiltrated all vertebral bodies, although the degree of involvement and the destruction of the outer contour are most marked at C2 and T1 in this example.

A gradient-recalled acquisition in steady state (GRASS) technique can accentuate the T1- and T2-weighted images in a relatively short time. By manipulation of the physical factors of the angle of proton spin, we can increase the sensitivity or conspicuity of the infiltrative pattern seen in the vertebral bodies. Note again that C2 and C7 are replaced by metastatic disease, but that a similar signal change is identified in all the other vertebral bodies included in the image (small arrows).

The extraosseous extent of the soft tissue is also nicely evaluated with MRI. Go back and look at Figures 1 and 2. The open arrow demonstrates anterior spread of the tumor into the prevertebral soft tissues at the C2 level. Note the indentation into the air space just below the uvula (open arrows).

After investigating the primary area of interest (i.e., the vertebral body and cord), it is always valuable to go back and inspect the soft tissues and the areas that are not the main focus of any study.

9.23 EPIDURAL METASTATIC DISEASE INVOLVING THE C6 VERTEBRAL BODY

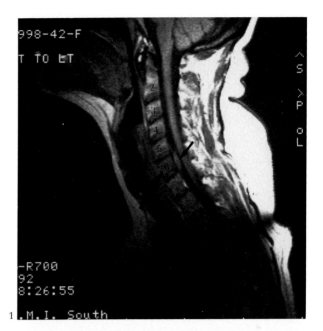

Figure 1 (large arrow) points to slight signal loss in the C6 vertebral body compared to C5 or C7 vertebral bodies. Additionally, note the nice demonstration of an epidural collection posterior to C6 that touches the cord (small arrow). This finding is typical of metastatic involvement of the vertebral body. The demonstration of epidural spread is also important, since it can be used to assess the pressure or absence of cord compression in the area of involvement.

Figure 2 (curved arrow) demonstrates the extension into the epidural space and neuroforaminal canal on the right side. Figure 3, a slightly lower cut, demonstrates the epidural spread as it extends into the canal and displaces the cord from right to left. Note that there is still visualization of CSF surrounding the cord, and that the cord is simply displaced, not compressed, at this level.

MRI is a painless and relatively brief exam (45–60 minutes) compared to the several hours that may be needed for a total myelogram in a patient with progressive neurological defect for screening and exclusion of cord compression.

One of the unique advantages of MRI is that there is no need to move or manipulate a patient with a questionable neurological deficit that may be progressive. I do not consider total body myelography to be a noninvasive study. In addition, the patient must be moved into several uncomfortable, if not inadvisable, positions, particularly when the upper cervical cord may be already at risk or impaired.

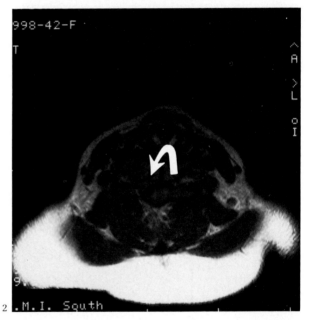

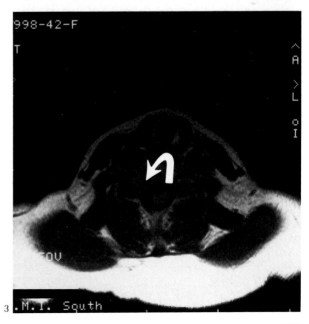

9.24 CERVICAL DISC HERNIATION

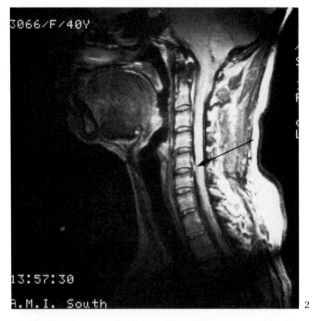

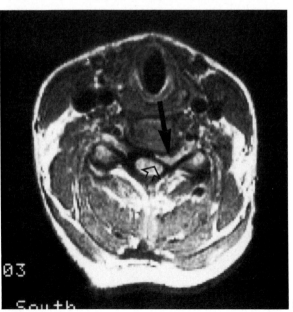

This is a typical example of a cervical herniation. The patient is 40 years old. The disc herniation can be characterized as either predominantly soft or composed mainly of annular and nuclear pulposa material. Figure 1 (long-stemmed arrow) points to the defect, which extends posterior to the posterior vertebral body line and causes a slight mass effect upon the cord. Figure 2, a more proton density-weighted image, shows that a portion of this defect increased in signal. This may be difficult to separate completely from an abnormally distended epidural vein in the cervical region.

Figure 3 is a high-quality axial image that can be obtained routinely using today's software. The long-stemmed arrow demonstrates the herniated material extending into the left central and neuroforaminal canals.

The opened arrow in Figure 3 demonstrates the mass effect upon and flattening of the cord. At times, even when direct visualization on the axial image of the herniation is not possible, the presence of cord flattening should suggest that a defect is present. Reexamination of the sagittal images will usually yield proof of such a defect.

At the time of this writing, contrast CT followed by myelography was believed to be the most sensitive axial imaging parameter for detection of herniation. However, with the images submitted here, the detection of herniation should favor MRI, since both sagittal and axial images are used. MRI is seldom compared as a whole exam to the CT studies in the current literature. The tendency has been to compare axial MRI to the axial CT. I think that at this time MRI is close, if not ready, to surpass CT even in the axial area only. However, MRI should be regarded as a study in its entirety; the sagittal images yield an additional increase in sensitivity for the detection of herniation. They also cover a larger area of the cervical spine, typically including the area from the base of the foramen magnum to at least T2 on almost every machine used and in all but the largest body habituses encountered in the clinical setting. Up to recently, most institutions used CT only from about the C4–5 through the C7–T1 level, which overlooks C2–3 and C3–4 unless accompanied by myelography-directed techniques. MRI typically can include all of this area, as well as the upper thoracic regions.

9.25 SMALL CERVICAL CORD SYRINX, POSSIBLY ASSOCIATED WITH TWO CERVICAL HERNIATIONS

Moderate-sized central herniations at the C5–6 and C6–7 levels are identified by the small arrows on Figure 1. Characteristic projection of nuclear material beyond the vertebral body end plates' more posterior aspect is identified. This causes a small amount of mass effect upon the cord at both levels. More interestingly in this case, caudal to these defects is a small syrinx within the cervical cord. The most cephalad area of the syrinx is identified with the long-stemmed arrows on Figure 1. With T2-weighted images, the syrinx may extend slightly higher (long-stemmed arrow, Figure 2). Figure 3, an axial image, verifies that this is truly a syrinx. This patient's images are high in quality, and none of the truncation artifact that can sometimes mimic a small syrinx is seen. No chemical shifting or other technical factors raise the suspicion that the syrinx is not real. However, the second view is always helpful in confirming the presence of a syrinx.

There is little in the literature to suggest the possible relationship, but it is possible that herniations may indent upon the cord and obstruct normal CSF pathways, allowing CSF to accumulate in the central canal region, as is seen here.

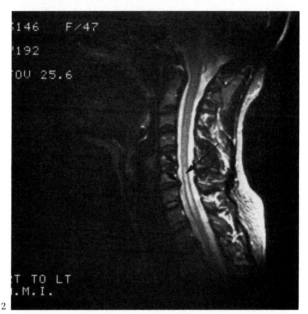

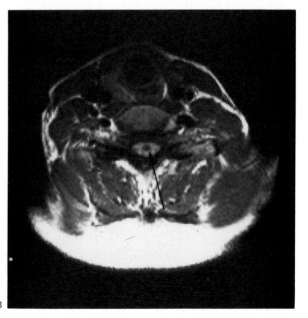

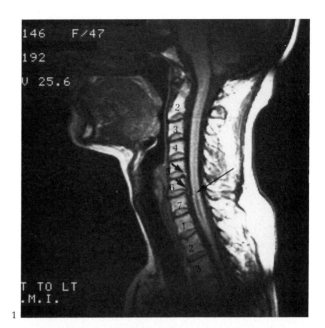

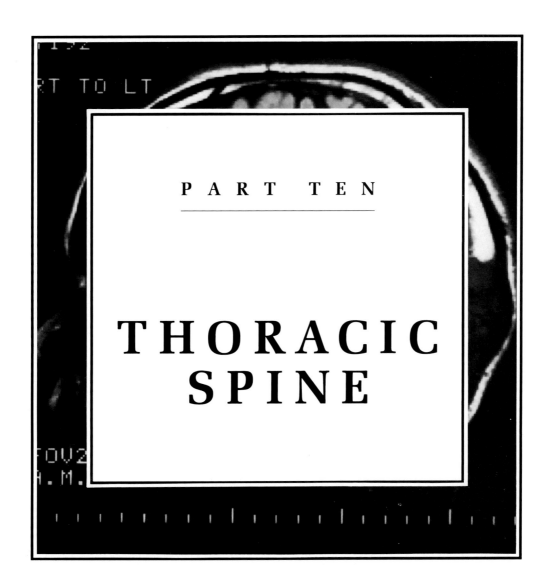

PART TEN

THORACIC SPINE

10.1 POSTERIOR SCAPULAR LIPOMA

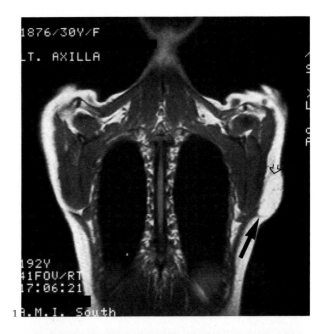

On Figure 1, note the presence of an asymmetric fatty mass posterior to the scapular muscles. The solid large arrow points to the inferior aspect of this mass, and the open arrowhead demonstrates its upper cranial extent. Figure 2 demonstrates the axial cut through this mass. The curved arrow points to the normal right side. Note the thin normal appearance of the subcutaneous tissue in contrast to the left side, where the open arrowheads point to the region of the exiting mass. In terms of signal intensity, the mass behaves similarly to the surrounding normal subcutaneous tissues. Figure 3, a T2-weighted image, verifies the presence of fatty material within this tumor. A small water bottle has been placed over the area of the perceptible mass for identification of the area in question (large white arrow). With MRI, detection of such incidental lipomas is much easier, and patients can be assured of the fatty nature of the tumor. With lipomas, however, caution must be used because any increased interstitial structure or solid tissue within the lipoma other than fat should raise the suspicion of possible underlying liposarcoma.

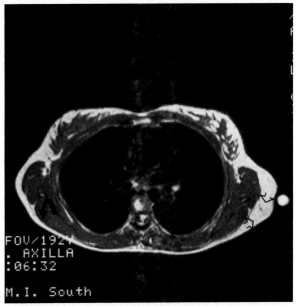

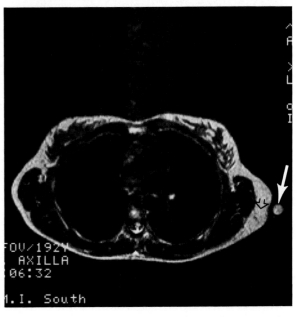

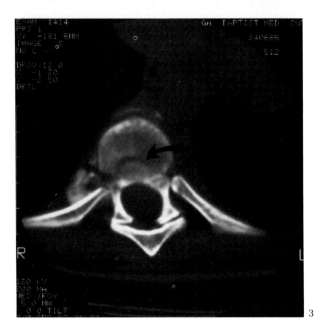

10.2 COMPRESSION OF CORD SECONDARY TO FRACTURE OF THORACIC VERTEBRAL BODY

Figure 1 is a scout film demonstrating compression, kyphotic angulation, and retropulsion of the vertebral body into the canal (large arrow). Note the narrowed appearance of the cord and the increased signal suggesting underlying edema. Note the normal appearance of the cord above and below the area of damage (arrowheads).

Figure 2 is an MRI scan of the axial cut through the level of compression. The defect can be identified (curved arrow), and the cord is flattened (open arrowhead). Figure 3, a CT cut through the same level, demonstrates a fracture through the vertebral body (curved arrow). However, note that the cord cannot be directly visualized despite changes in windowing and centering.

Figure 4 is a plain film demonstrating the compression fracture in the thoracic spine (large arrow).

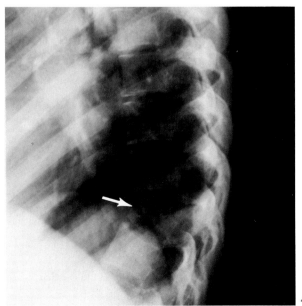

10.3 COMPRESSION FRACTURE OF THORACIC VERTEBRAL BODY

Figure 1 demonstrates marked compression of a thoracic vertebral body (curved arrow). A large fragment has been pushed into the canal (open arrowhead). Note the relationship of the fragment to the cord, which is compressed and deviated. Figure 2 is an axial cut through this same level demonstrating the bone fragment pushing into the thoracic cord (open arrowhead). The cord can also be visualized on the axial cut (small arrow).

This case is through the courtesy of Dr. Walter Bednarz of Williamsport Magnetic Imaging.

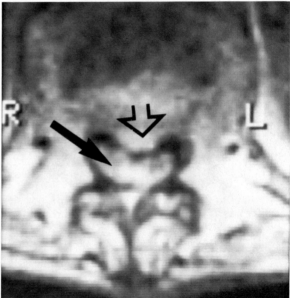

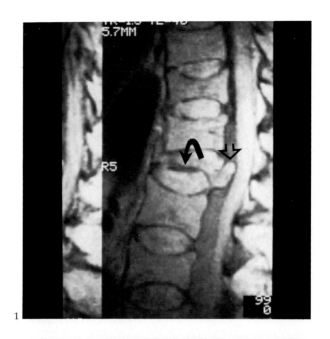

10.4 COMPRESSION FRACTURE AT T6 WITH A T1–2 DISC HERNIATION

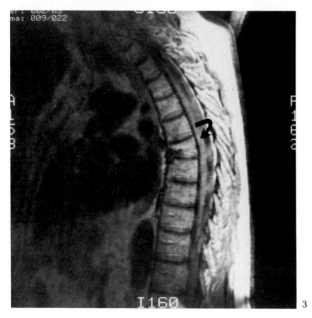

Figure 1 demonstrates herniations at the C5–6 and C6–7 levels. Also note the herniation present at T1–2 (arrowheads).

Figure 2 demonstrates compression of the T6 vertebral body (arrow). Note that the posterior aspect of the vertebral bodies is nicely identified, and the absence of cord compression can be verified (curved arrow, Figure 3). The thoracic vertebral bodies, like the lumbar spine, can be nicely evaluated with MRI for the detection of compression fracture. The relationship of the damaged vertebral body to the cord within the canal and for identification of disc herniations is demonstrated here. In many regards, MRI is a vastly improved screening modality compared to the thoracic myelogram. Thoracic myelography can be technically difficult and the coverage of the thoracic spine can vary widely, depending upon the radiologist's skills and the patient's body habitus.

10.5 THORACIC HERNIATION

The same criteria used for herniations in the lumbar region apply to the thoracic spine. A cranially migrated fragment from a T5–6 disc herniation is demonstrated on Figure 1 (large arrow). The defect can again be confirmed on the T2-weighted images at this same level (Figure 2, large arrow). Axial images can also demonstrate the relationship of the extradural defect, as seen on Figure 3a, and interface with the thoracic cord and the amount of cord compression can be documented (long-stemmed arrow).

Figure 3b is the cut immediately below, again demonstrating the extradural defect (open arrowhead). Note again the compression of the thoracic cord.

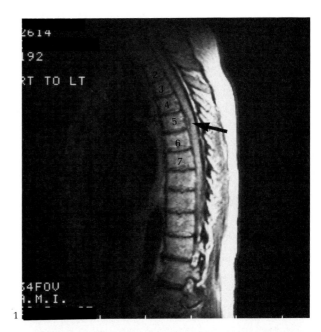

1

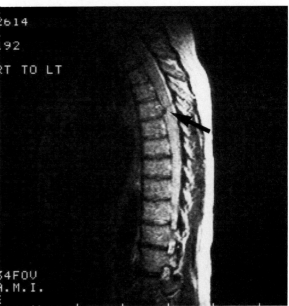

2

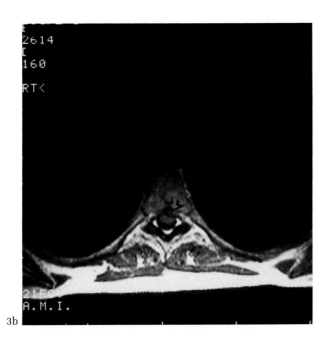

3b

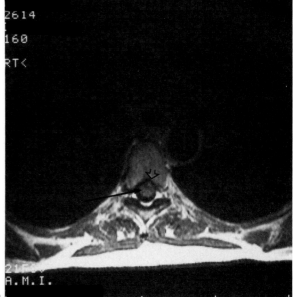

3a

10.6 GUNSHOT INJURY TO THE THORACIC CORD

Figure 1 demonstrates the irregular appearance of the mid-thoracic cord between the relatively normal superior and inferior segments (arrows). There has been a gunshot injury to the thoracic spine, and a large posterior hematoma is also identified (curved arrows).

Figure 2 is a T2-weighted sagittal cut through this same level. The arrowhead points to an area of increased signal where the normal cord parenchyma should exist, reflecting CSF behavior in this region rather than cord signal intensity. Incidentally, note that the hematoma now seen on the T2-weighted images is dark (curved arrows).

Figure 3, an axial cut through the area of maximal damage, demonstrates only a small wafer of residual neural tissue (arrow). Figure 4, a cut just inferior to Figure 3, demonstrates a more normal cord, but the cord size is atrophic secondary to degeneration following severe trauma to this structure.

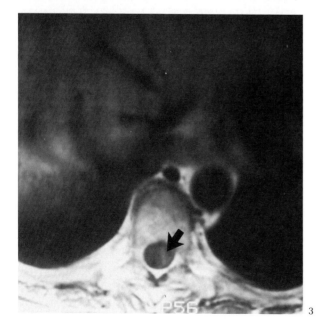

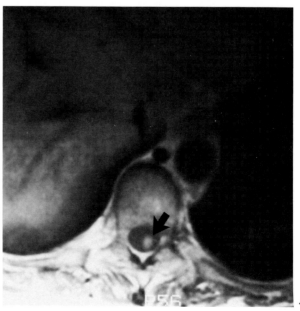

10.7 SEVERE CYSTIC MYELOMALACIA FOLLOWING GUNSHOT INJURY

Figures 1 and 2 demonstrate marked cystic myelomalacia. Figure 1 (solid arrow) demonstrates the cord as it is separated by the degenerative cyst; the open arrowhead points to an area of cystic change in the traumatized cord. Figure 2 (curved arrow) points to some of the septations in the area of cystic myelomalacia; the arrowhead points to the small atrophic but intact superior cord above the level of damage. As with all injuries, whether blunt or secondary to high-velocity missile damage, MRI is uniquely suited to direct visualization of the cord. The later sequelae, such as the cystic myelomalacia demonstrated here, can also be followed, and the evolution of cyst and damage within the cord can be monitored for possible surgical intervention to prevent further neurological loss in the follow-up of such trauma patients.

This case is through the courtesy of Dr. Jack Greenberg of Philadelphia Magnetic Imaging.

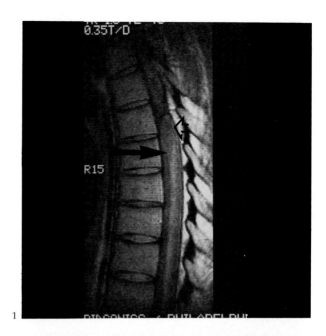

1

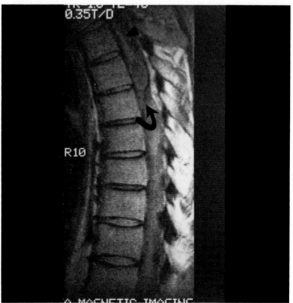

2

10.8 SINGLE MS PLAQUE IN THE THORACIC CORD

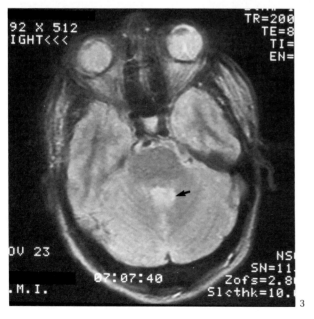

Figure 1 demonstrates an irregular, flame-shaped area of increased signal in the thoracic cord (arrow). This correlates with subtle findings of MS in the cranium on Figures 2 and 3. Paraventricular areas of increased signal can be identified (arrows).

The association of intracranial MS with the spine is known; approximately 10 percent of the lesions can be found in the spinal cord. They are usually not isolated in the cord. A cranial study should accompany or, preferably, precede investigation of the spinal cord in a patient suspected of having MS.

10.9 MS INVOLVEMENT OF THE THORACIC CORD

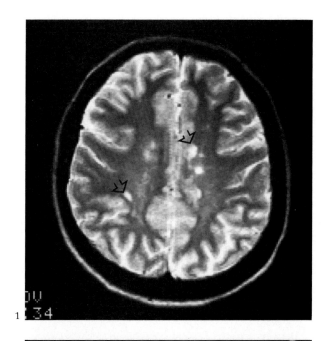

Figure 1 demonstrates the typical white matter lesions consistent with the diagnosis of MS. Figure 2 demonstrates a typical flame-shaped area of plaque involving the upper cervical cord at the C2–3 level. An additional area of involvement was found with scanning of the thoracic cord at the T6 and T8–9 levels. The flame-shaped areas of increased signal can be identified on Figure 3a (arrows). They are somewhat less easily identified in this particular example on the T2-weighted images (Figure 3b); usually the T2-weighted images are more helpful in detecting the regions of plaque (arrows). The thoracic cord can be involved with MS, and if the findings in a patient suspected of having MS are not explained satisfactorily with the cranial investigation, the spinal cord should be evaluated as well. We begin all suspected MS workup with the cranial investigation, followed by assessment of the spinal cord.

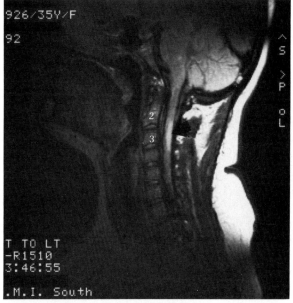

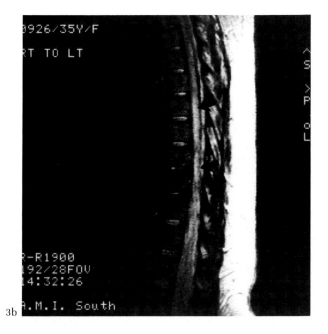

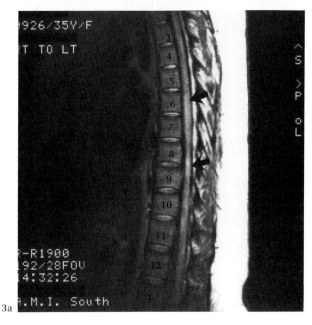

10.10 ADRENAL CANCER METASTASIS TO THE THORACIC SPINE WITH CORD COMPRESSION

The T3 vertebral body is almost completely compressed, and there is evidence of high-grade cord compression on Figure 1 (large arrow). This is a body scout image for purposes of counting. It is always necessary to include an anatomic landmark such as the C1–2 junction for certainty in counting for levels of involvement.

Figure 2 is a routine surface coil image demonstrating the large epidural mass compressing the cord (small arrow). The degree of cord compression is nicely illustrated (large arrow). T3 is now almost entirely flattened and wafer thin (curved arrow). Figure 3 is an axial cut through this level of compression demonstrating the marked vertebral body destruction and the extraosseous spread of tumor (large arrow). The canal has been markedly compromised (arrowhead). Incidental note is also made of a malignant effusion in the right pleural space (open arrowhead).

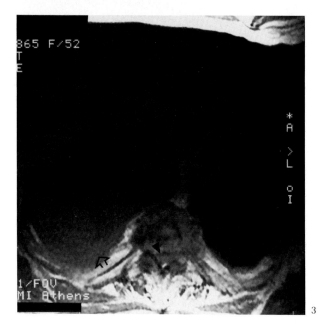

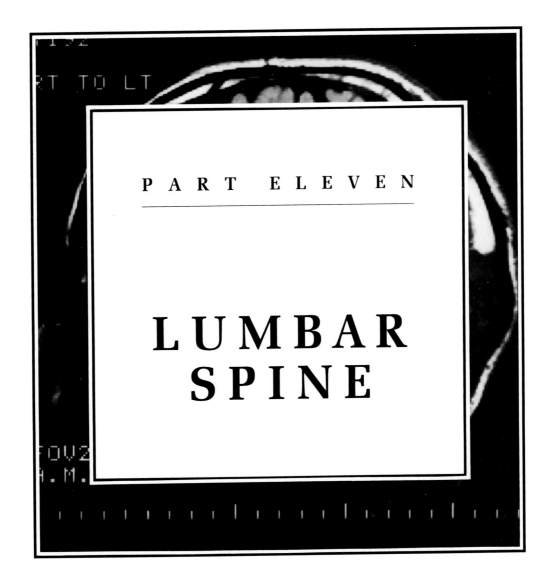

PART ELEVEN

LUMBAR SPINE

11.1 SMALL CSF LEAK FOLLOWING BACK SURGERY

Figure 1 demonstrates the absence of the spine and the presence of a small left laminectomy. However, a tract of CSF intensity is seen exiting from the posterior aspect of the canal (long-stemmed arrows). To the left of the midline is a high-signal, lens-shaped collection (small arrows); this is consistent with a small amount of hematoma, which is now old.

Figure 2 is an axial image above the level of the leak showing the postsurgical pseudomeningocele (large arrow).

Figure 3 is a sagittal view of this collection extending from the operative site to a position at the level of the lower thoracic spine. The small arrows demonstrate the interface between the pseudomeningocele and the subcutaneous fat.

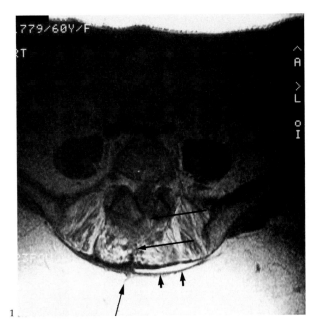

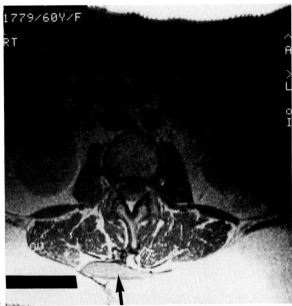

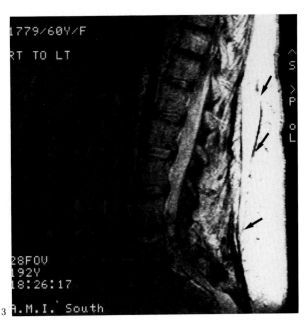

11.2 LAMINECTOMY DEFECT WITH LARGE HERNIATION

Figure 1a demonstrates a herniation on a T1-weighted sagittal image (curved arrow). Figure 1b is a T2-weighted image demonstrating the herniation. Note the elevation of the posterior longitudinal ligament (arrowheads). Figure 2 demonstrates the large left central herniation (large arrows). The interface between the disc herniation and the thecal sac can be identified (small arrows).

Figure 3 demonstrates the absence of the lamina on the right side (large arrow). Note that this is now filled in with high-signal fat. Compare this to the normal-appearing lamina on the left side (curved arrow).

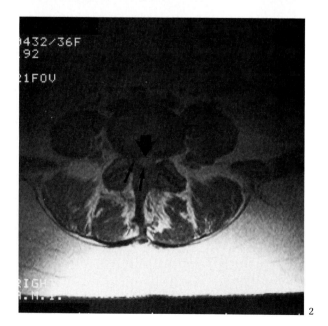

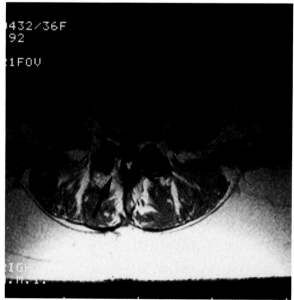

11.3 POST-OPERATIVE SCARRING

Figures 1 and 2 demonstrate a sheet-like area of irregular intermediate signal posterior to the L5 vertebral body and extending up to the L4–5 disc space (large arrows). Note that the annular defect can be identified (long-stemmed arrow). There is absence of bone posterior to the L5 level correlating with a laminectomy defect (arrowhead). Figure 3 demonstrates the laminectomy defect (large arrow). Figure 4 demonstrates the exiting L4 rootlets (small arrows) and again confirms the absence of the lamina on the right side (large arrow).

Prior to the development of Magnevist, scar tissue was identified on MRI scans as having an irregular, sheet-like appearance. There was a lack of mass effect, and no focal nidus of herniation could be identified within the scar tissue. With Magnevist this differentiation is less necessary, and postoperative examination of the back, primarily to distinguish herniation from scar tissue, should not be performed with Magnevist.

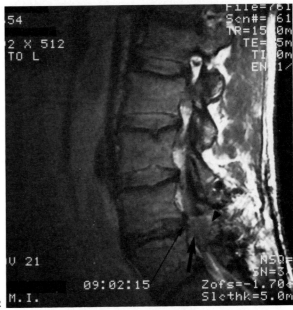

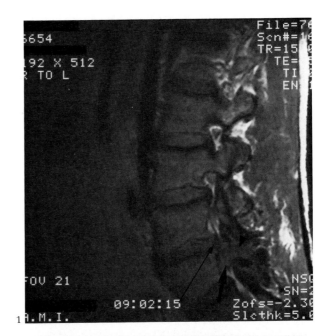

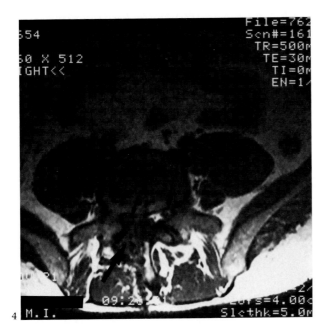

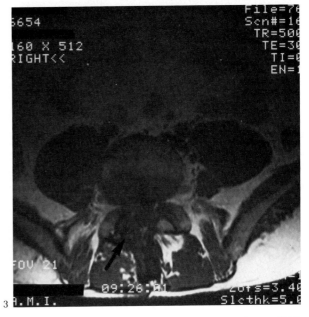

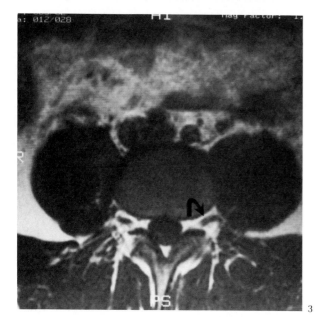

11.4 MAGNEVIST-ENHANCED RECURRENT HERNIATION AT L5–S1

Figure 1 is a nonenhanced study at the L5–S1 level. The defect can be seen (curved arrow). The interface between the thecal sac is subtle but present (small arrow).

Figure 2 is a Magnevist injection and repeat study at the same level. The S1 root, which is swollen and deviated posteriorly, is now identified (large arrow). The defect is not enhancing (curved arrows), but there is enhancement surrounding the defect and the root (small arrows). Figure 3a is a nonenhanced axial cut through an upper normal level. Note the exiting nerve root (curved arrow). With Magnevist no enhancement of scar tissue is seen, and the epidural fat and structures are as seen on Figure 3b. The exiting root is again identified with the curved arrow.

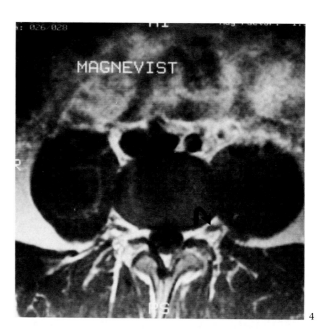

11.5 CONUS TUMOR, LIPOMA VERSUS DERMOID

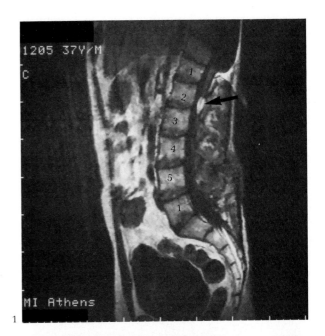
1

Figure 1 is a scout film demonstrating a high signal intensity in the region of the conus (large arrow). Figure 2 is a routine surface coil image demonstrating again a well-circumscribed, high signal intensity structure (large arrow). Figure 3 is a T2-weighted image in which the tumor now blends with the increased signal intensity of the CSF.

Increased signal and tumors in the lumbar spine usually reflect a high lipid content; this is consistent with lipoma or dermoid. The detection of conus tumors and tumors in the upper lumbar spine can be useful. As stated earlier, routine CT scanning of the lumbar spine usually does not include the L1–2 level.

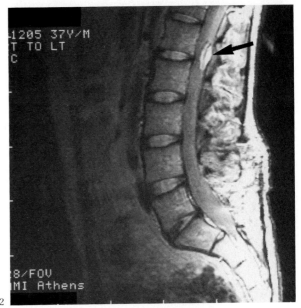
2

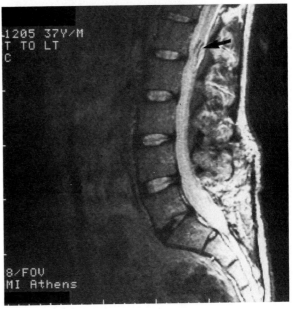
3

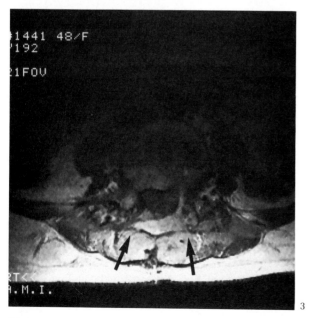

11.6 MARKED L4–5 SUBLUXATION WITH CANAL STENOSIS

Figure 1 demonstrates anterior subluxation of L4 on L5 (large arrow). Note the disintegration and narrowing of the L4–5 disc space, with material included within the still intact posterior annulus (arrowhead). Note that the canal is markedly stenotic at this level (small arrow). Figure 2 is a T2-weighted image through this same cut. The myelographic effect now demonstrates the striking loss of space at the L4–5 level secondary to this degenerative slippage.

This patient has been treated with fusion, which is identified nicely in the axial plane (Figure 3, large arrows). Inspection of the fusion masses for pseudoarthrosis with MRI is useful. This fusion appears intact and solid.

11.7 GRADE I SPONDYLOLISTHESIS

Figure 1 is a sagittal cut demonstrating the slippage of L5 on the S1 vertebral body (large arrow). The small arrow demonstrates, in the sagittal plane, a defect or cleft through the pars intra-articularis consistent with spondylosis. The association of the slippage and the defect in the pars intra-articularis is referred to as *spondylolisthesis*. There can be several grades of spondylolisthesis, depending on the amount of slippage of L5 on S1. Figure 2 is an axial cut demonstrating the pars defects in the axial plane (curved arrows). Incidentally note that, because of flowing blood, the epidural veins are present with a signal void and can be isolated within the high-signal epidural fat at this level (long-stemmed arrow).

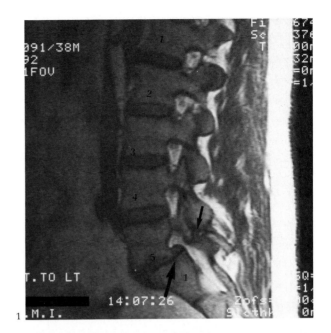

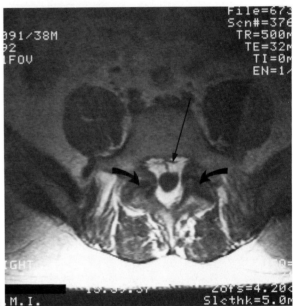

11.8 L4–5 STENOSIS SECONDARY TO FACET HYPERTROPHY

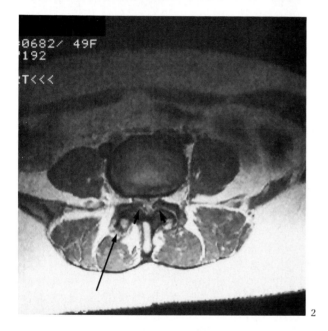

1

Figure 1 demonstrates a large posterior defect compressing and narrowing the lumbar canal at the L4–5 level (large arrow). Figure 2 is an axial cut demonstrating the hypertrophied appearance of the facets anteriorly (small arrows). Some ligamentous hypertrophy is also present. Note that the bony hypertrophy on the right is also pronounced posteriorly (long-stemmed arrows).

Figure 1 also demonstrates the presence of some degenerative anterior slippage of L4 on L5 and a diffuse bulge of the annulus at the L4–5 level (long-stemmed arrow). This contributes to the stenosis seen; however, the posterior element hypertrophy is predominantly responsible for the stenosis.

Figure 3 is a normal axial cut through the facets at the normal level in the same patient. The highland cartilage of the facets can be identified (small arrows). Note the normal appearance of the facets in regard to bony overgrowth (long-stemmed arrow). Also note that the ligamentum flavum can be identified separately from the cortical line of the facets and the thecal sac (curved arrow).

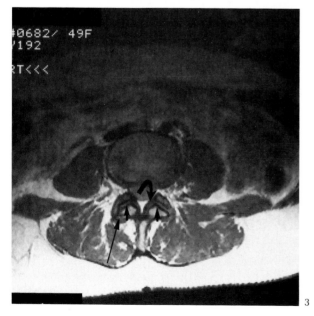

3

310

11.9 CONJOINED ROOTS

Figure 1 demonstrates expansion of the normal left neuroforaminal canal at the L4–5 level (open arrowhead). Figure 2 demonstrates the separation of the nerve roots as they exit through the neuroforaminal canal (large arrowhead).

Figure 3 is a sagittal cut through the exiting conjoined roots (curved arrow).

The bony enlargement in the superolateral recess demonstrates the long-term presence of this condition and is evidence against malignant change. A similar bony expansion can be associated with neurofibroma. However, the sagittal images did not detect the presence of an enhancing lesion in this region. Figure 2 demonstrates the separating roots as they exit through the left-sided neuroforaminal canal. Conjoint root is a congenital variation and should not be confused with a tumor or significant abnormality.

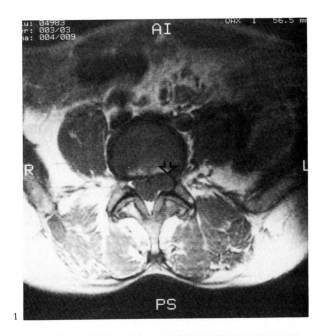

1

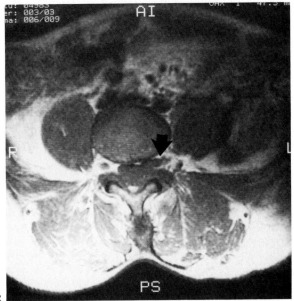

2

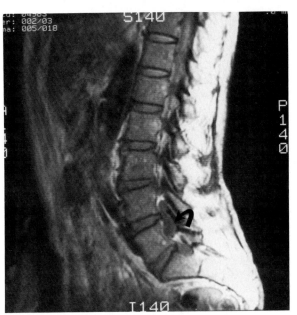

3

11.10 FACET SYNOVIAL CYST

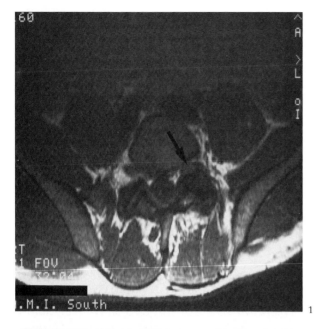

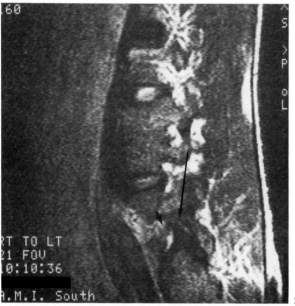

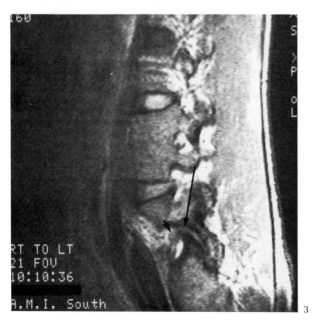

Figure 1 demonstrates a small mass arising from the anterior aspect of the facet (large arrow). The long-stemmed arrows in Figures 2 and 3 point to the joint space of the facet, and the small arrow points to the cyst in continuity with the joint space. The posterior elements can undergo degenerative changes. These synovial cysts are quite similar to synovial cysts seen in other articular surfaces, the most well known being the knee.

11.11 L4–5 DISC HERNIATION

Figure 1 demonstrates the typical appearance of a large herniation (large arrow). Note that the annulus has been torn (arrowhead). The posterior longitudinal ligament has also been elevated secondary to this herniation (small arrow). Figure 2 is an axial cut through this level. The large arrow points to the herniated material. The outer contour of this material can be identified as a low-density line (long-stemmed arrow). Figure 3 is a T2-weighted image through the herniation. The herniation is again identified (curved arrow). The open arrowhead points to a slight increase in signal in the epidural space above and below the defect. This signal is higher than that of the fat at this level and probably represents distention of epidural veins.

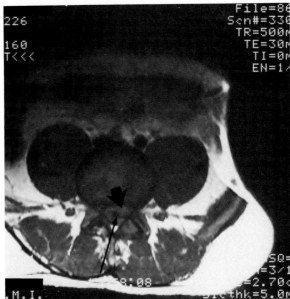

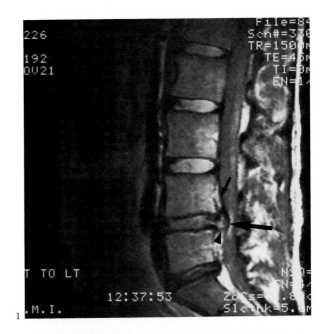

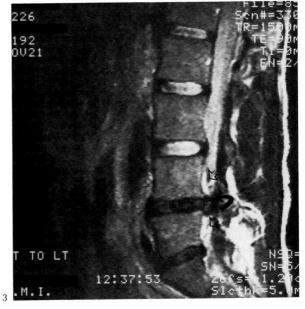

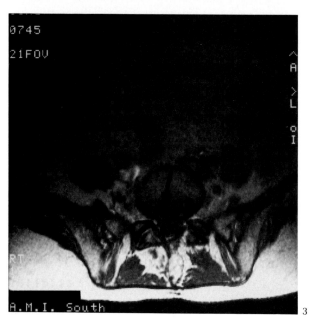

11.12 RIGHT-SIDED L5–S1 HERNIATION WITH CEPHALAD MIGRATION OF A FRAGMENT

Figure 1 demonstrates herniation at the L5–S1 level (large arrow). Note that the fragment has extended cephalad. Figure 2 is a T2-weighted image through this same level. Go back to Figure 1 and note the degenerative appearance of the L4–5 disc (open arrowheads). The posterior annulus at this level is intact, and no extradural defect at any other level can be seen.

Figure 3 is an axial cut through the level of the herniation (large arrow).

The ability to demonstrate not only herniation but also its relationship to the vertebral bodies allows more complete decompression and prevents retention of free fragments intraoperatively.

11.13 L4–5 DISC BULGE

Figure 1 demonstrates a right-sided parasagittal cut; the bulge can be identified (large arrow). Note that it touches the exiting L3 root (curved arrow); however, the root is still surrounded by epidural fat. Figure 2 is an axial cut at the same level as the CT scan on Figure 3. The large arrow points to the defect on the right at the L4–5 level. The maintenance of a normal low-signal rim of annular fiber allows the diagnosis of annulur bulging rather than frank herniation.

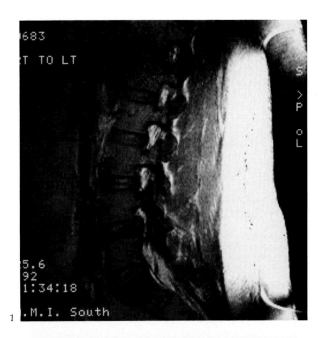

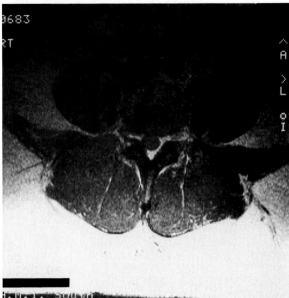

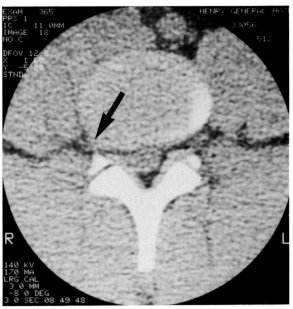

11.14 LARGE L5–S1 DISC HERNIATION

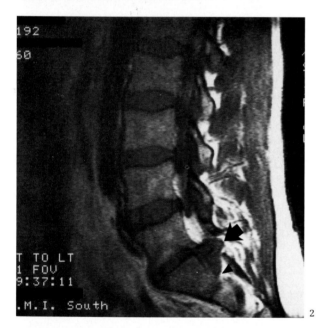

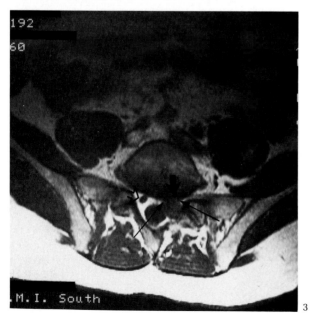

1

2

3

Figures 1 and 2 are parasagittal cuts through a disc herniation at the L5–S1 level (large arrows). The cleft in the annulus can be nicely identified on Figure 1 (long-stemmed arrow). The caudal extent of this caudally migrated material is identified by the arrowheads.

Figure 3 identifies the herniation in the axial plane (large arrow). The break in the annulus and its continuity with the herniated material can be identified (long-stemmed arrow). The exiting S1 root on the left is compressed and invisible on this image. Note the normal appearance of the exiting right-sided S1 root (open arrowhead). It is a low-density structure surrounded by high signal from the normal epidural fat surrounding the rootlet.

11.15 THE IMPORTANCE OF THE PARASAGITTAL AND AXIAL IMAGES IN THE DETECTION OF HERNIATIONS

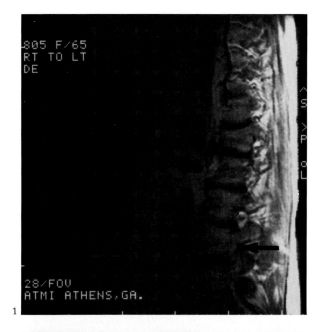

1

Figure 1 (large arrow) points to a disc herniation that has migrated into the neuroforaminal canal (large arrow); compare the neuroforaminal canals above and below (open arrowhead). Note that the nerve roots and vessels are surrounded by more high-signal epidural fat. Also note that the annulus is breached by a tear represented by a cleft in the normally low-signal annulus (long-stemmed arrow). Figure 2 is an axial view confirming the presence of a disc herniation (large arrow).

In fairness to the sagittal cuts, the T2-weighted images do show the defect (curved arrow, Figure 3a). However, it may be overlooked without the clue provided by the parasagittal cuts.

Incidental note is made of the appearance of an old flexion compression fracture of the L1 vertebral body on the T2-weighted image (Figure 3a) and the T1-weighted image (Figure 3b). This case is a reminder that the more extreme parasagittal cuts can be very valuable and that inspection of the normal epidural fat in the neuroforaminal canals should be an important routine portion of the evaluation of the lumbar spine. Additionally, it is essential to always include axial images when studying a portion of the spine. Axial images prevent underestimation of disc herniation.

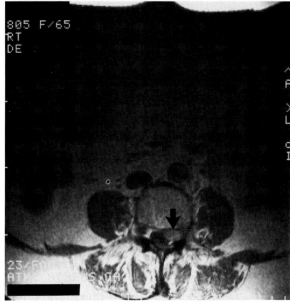

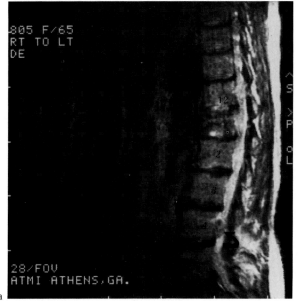

2

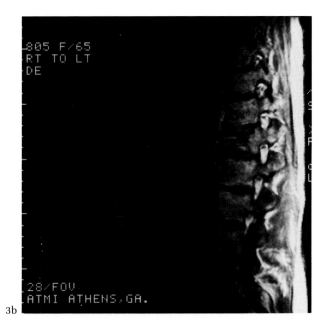

3b

3a

11.16 RIGHT-SIDED L5–S1 HERNIATION

Figures 1a and 1b show the T1- and T2-weighted appearance of a double-echo sagittal study demonstrating a herniation (large arrows). Note that most of the herniation is contained within the insensitive epidural fat, which can normally be increased in width at the L5–S1 level (arrowheads). A lateral myelographic finding may totally miss the presence of a large defect here because the thecal sac would not be impressed upon. Figure 2 is a more sagittal cut demonstrating the large amount of herniated material (arrows) to the right of midline. Figure 3 is an axial cut demonstrating the compression of the root, which would be detected on the lateral and anteroposterior views even on myelography (curved arrow). Note the S1 root on the left as it exits the thecal sac (arrowhead).

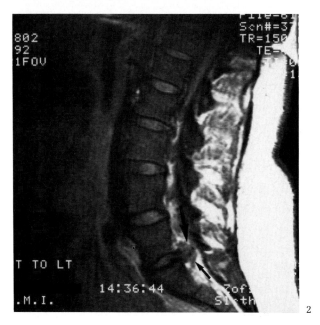

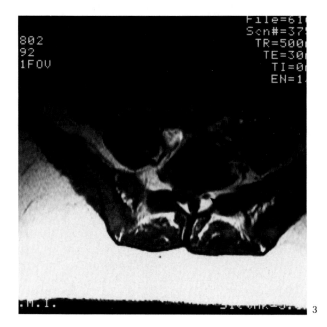

11.17 L1–2 DISC HERNIATION WITH CONUS COMPRESSION

Figure 1 demonstrates a herniation at the L1–2 level (large arrow). Note that the conus can be identified (curved arrow). Figure 2 is a T2-weighted image again identifying the defect at the L1–2 level (large arrow).

Figure 3 demonstrates the relationship of the conus (small arrow) to the extradural defect (curved arrow).

This case is important in that the usual coverage of the lumbar spine with CT typically includes the L3–4 through L5–S1 levels; the lower thoracic and upper lumbar spines are usually not included in a screening exam. MRI shows great promise in including T12 through S1, thereby allowing evaluation of more disc levels. Some of the old statistics about the frequency of disc herniations may be revised as a result of this new imaging modality.

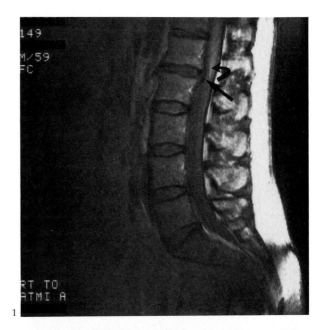

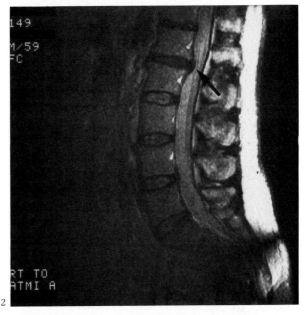

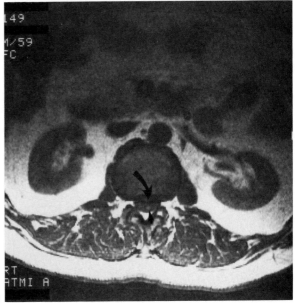

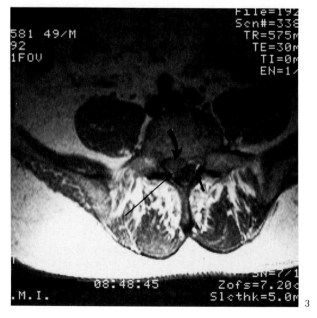

11.18 L4–5 DISC HERNIATION WITH CAUDAL MIGRATION OF A FRAGMENT

Figure 1 demonstrates a large herniation that has extended caudally from the L4–5 disc. Figure 2 demonstrates this herniation with a slight increase in signal (large arrow). Figure 3 is an axial cut demonstrating the large right-sided herniation and the normal appearance of the exiting root from the anterior thecal sac on the left (small arrow). Note that the interface between the thecal sac and the extradural defect can be identified (long-stemmed arrow).

11.19 MASSIVE L5–S1 HERNIATION, COMPARISON OF CT AND MRI

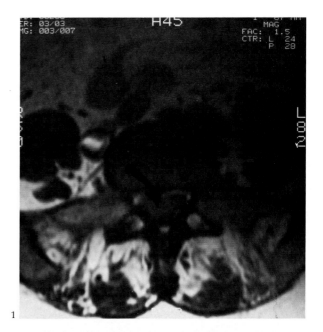

1

Figure 1 (curved arrow) points to a high-signal structure occupying almost the entire canal at the L5 level. Figure 2 is a CT cut through the same level demonstrating, less conspicuously, the presence of this large, herniated disc. The cut just above this on the study demonstrated right-sided herniation, although the size of the herniation was unchanged at the upper level. The presence of a large amount of material within the canal at this level was entirely missed by CT. Figure 3a is the sagittal representation of this herniation in its caudal extent (arrowhead). Figure 3b is a T2-weighted image. Note that the large herniated fragment can still be identified, but it now demonstrates an increased signal and almost blends with the CSF (arrowheads).

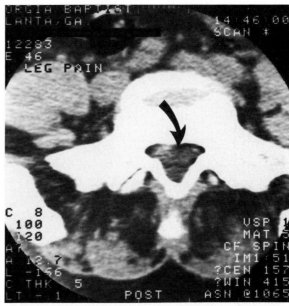

2

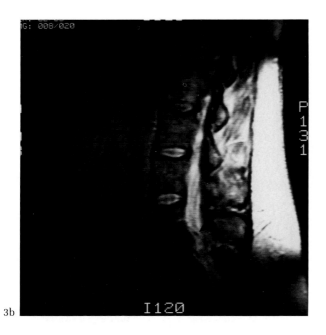

3b

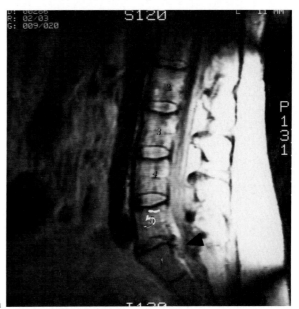

3a

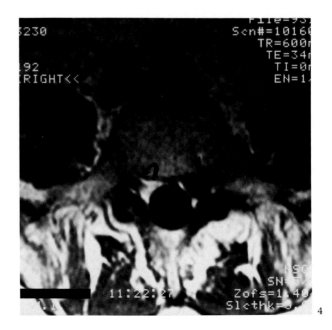

11.20 L4–5 HERNIATION WITH A CAUDAL FRAGMENT MIGRATING INTO THE NEUROFORAMINAL CANAL

Figure 1 demonstrates a defect in the annulus at the L4–5 level, but no significant extradural defect can be identified (small arrow). Figure 2 demonstrates, caudal to the L4–5 disc, the presence of a large fragment. When the contiguous sagittal structures were combined, this fragment seemed to be confluent with the L4–5 level. Figure 3 is an axial image demonstrating the small central defect (small arrow) at the L4–5 level. Figure 4, at the L5 level, demonstrates the replacement of epidural fat in the neuroforaminal canal secondary to a migrating disc fragment. Note the normal appearance of the superior-lateral recess at this level on the right (curved arrow).

11.21 MASSIVE L4–5 DISC HERNIATION

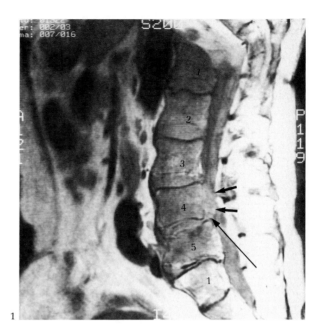

Figure 1 demonstrates diffuse signal loss of the L1 through L5 vertebral bodies. In addition, a large cranially directed extradural defect is seen posterior to the entire length of the L4 vertebral body (arrows). There is direct visualization of the annular tear, which allows a confident diagnosis of disc herniation (long-stemmed arrow). The axial cut on Figure 2 demonstrates the extensive amount of material herniating into the spinal canal and compressing the thecal sac (large arrows demonstrate the anterior and posterior extents of the herniation).

Figure 3, for comparative purposes, is the CT scan done at the same time. Note its relative inability to identify the extradural defect and its relationship to the thecal sac without thecal contrast.

At the time, this CT scan provided a diagnostic dilemma. Because of the loss of signal in the presence of an epidural mass, concern about underlying malignancy or infection was raised. However, operative decompression of the herniated material and biopsy of the vertebral bodies yielded no tumor. The decrease in signal was believed to represent increased cellularity in the bone marrow. Recent literature suggests that reactivated bone marrow can demonstrate decreased signal secondary to the increase in bone marrow-making cells, which replace the fatty components. This does not mean that focal low-signal areas in vertebral bodies can be ignored, but the recent finding of reactivated bone marrow has certainly made the differential diagnosis more difficult.

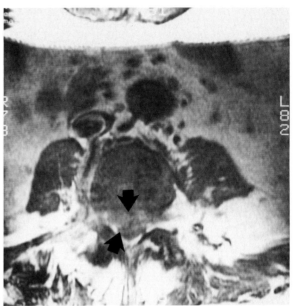

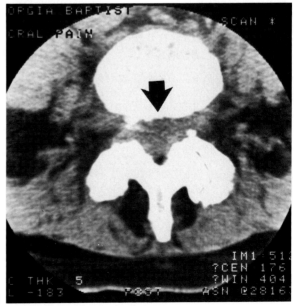

11.22 LARGE L5–S1 DISC HERNIATION WITH CAUDAL MIGRATION OF MATERIAL

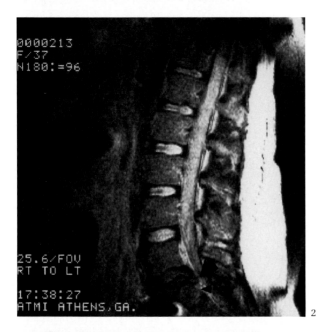

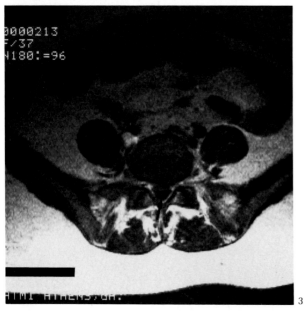

Figure 1 demonstrates a large extradural defect posterior to S1 (large arrow). Note also the tear through the annulus (long-stemmed arrow). The arrowhead points to the most caudal extent of the herniated material.

Figure 2 demonstrates the same findings on the T2-weighted image at the same level on the double-echo study. Figure 3 is an axial cut demonstrating the defect (open arrow) and its relationship to the thecal sac (small arrow).

The use of MRI makes the diagnosis of cephalad or cranially directed fragments quite easy; earlier, a slightly more rigorous thought process was required when clinicians were limited to simple axial CT scans. The extent of disc migration from the area of herniation can be important, and extensive herniations may require greater surgical exposure than a non-migrated herniation.

11.23 L4–5 DISC HERNIATION WITH INCREASED SIGNAL IN THE HERNIATED PORTION

Figure 1 is a T2-weighted image; there is increased signal in the herniated portion (large arrow). The increased signal can also be observed on the more T1-weighted image in the double-echo series (Figure 2, large arrow). The appearance of disc herniations can be quite varied, and it is essential to demonstrate the anatomy of the herniation in relation to the thecal sac. The signal characteristics can be quite misleading if one assumes that herniations emit only low signal. In particular, free fragments often demonstrate a marked increase in signal.

Figure 3 (large arrow) points to the disc herniation, which is slightly higher in signal than the thecal sac (open arrow).

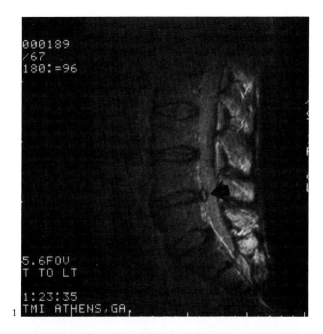

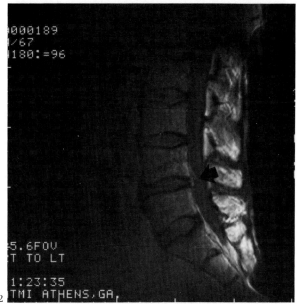

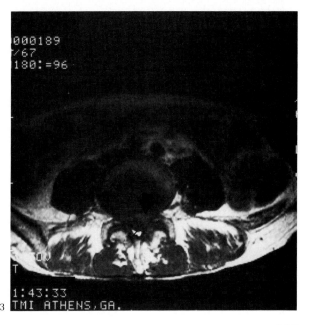

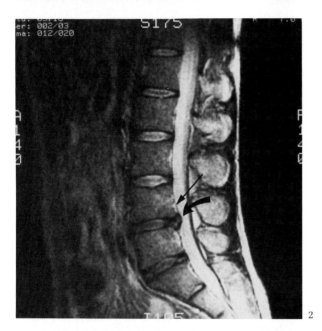

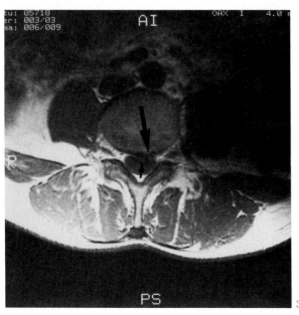

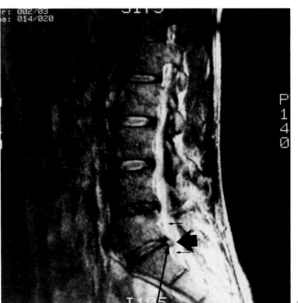

Figure 1 demonstrates the typical appearance of a small herniation at the L4–5 level (curved arrow). Note that the material extends posterior to the disc. On Figure 2 (curved arrow) the annulus appears thinned, if not torn. There also appears to be elevation of the posterior longitudinal ligament (long-stemmed arrow). Figure 3 demonstrates the herniation in the axial plane (large arrow). Note that the interface between the herniation and the thecal sac (small arrow) can be identified.

Figure 4 demonstrates an additional herniation at the L5–S1 level (large arrow). The nuclear material can be seen projecting beyond the posterior aspect of the vertebral bodies. In addition, the normal low-signal posterior annulus is absent, consistent with a tear in the annulus (long-stemmed arrow), and the tiny arrows demonstrate rootlets that are displaced by the herniation. MRI scanning of the lumbo-sacral spine should be the primary investigative tool when herniation is suspected. Its increased sensitivity and ability to examine this body part in more than one plane allow increased sensitivity and specificity with regard to herniated discs.

11.25 LATERAL HERNIATION AT THE L5–S1 LEVEL

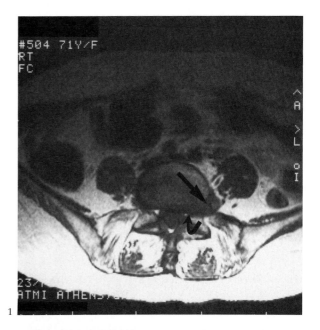

1

Figure 1 demonstrates a lateral herniated disc (large arrow). The importance of obtaining at least two views of any body part is well demonstrated by this case. Note that Figure 2, a routine central sagittal cut, fails to demonstrate any significant extradural defect. There is some signal loss reflecting degenerative change, and some anterior bulging of the disc is identified at this level. However, no significant posterior defect extending into the canal can be seen.

On an extreme level parasagittal cut (Figure 3), a suggestion of abnormality is seen (curved arrow). The annulus still appears to be intact, and a bulging disc posterior to the annulus can be visualized.

Such lateral herniations can be clinically significant, and inspection of the lateral and anterior portions of the disc in the study is very helpful. Often these lateral herniations are undetected on standard myelograms. Their significance has been better recognized with the advent of CT. It is hoped that now, with the use of MRI, the clinically significant lateral disc can be identified even more effectively. On Figure 1, note that the herniation also involves a large portion of the left neuroforaminal canal at this level (curved arrow).

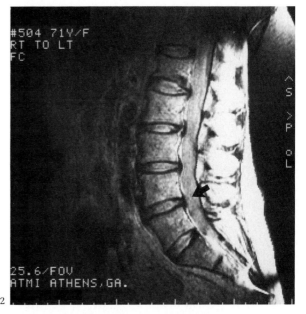

2

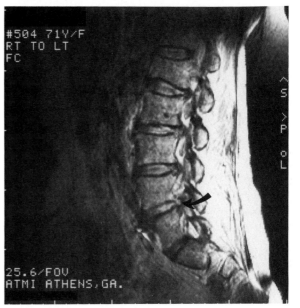

3

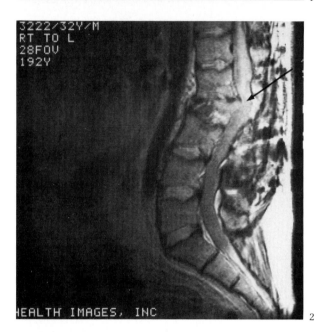

1

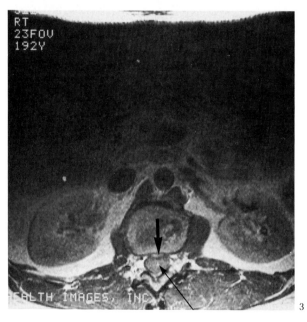

2

11.26 CANAL STENOSIS SECONDARY TO VERTEBRAL BODY FRACTURE AND RETROPULSION OF VERTEBRAL BODY FRAGMENTS

Figure 1 demonstrates marked fracture of the L2 vertebral body. There is retropulsion of the posterior superior end plate of L2 into the canal (long-stemmed arrow). Note also that the L1–2 and L2–3 discs have lost their normal signal, which reflects posttraumatic degenerative changes (arrowheads).

Figure 2 is a proton density image again demonstrating the defect at the L2 level. Note the ability to evaluate the vertebral bodies above and below the level of damage.

Figure 3 is an axial cut through a portion of the defect (large arrow). Note that the defect in relation to the canal can be identified. The solitary high signal intensity represents the filum (long-stemmed arrow).

3

11.27 LARGE L4–5 HERNIATION SIMULATING AN EPIDURAL TUMOR

Figure 1 demonstrates a degenerative disc at the L4–5 and L5–S1 levels. The arrowhead shows the annulus to be protruding but intact. The large arrow points to the large epidural mass that spans the L4–5 and L5–S1 levels. The curved arrow points to the posterior aspect of this mass, which extends through a significant portion of the canal. Figure 2 is a slightly more central sagittal cut, and the defect is again identified (large arrow). The small-stemmed arrow now demonstrates a breaker tear in the annulus, and the material in the epidural space communicates with that of the L4–5 disc. Also, go back to Figure 1 and note that the L4–5 disc is very narrowed. In addition, a typical Schmorl's node defect is seen in the inferior anterior end plate at L4 (open arrow).

Figure 3 is an axial cut demonstrating the extensive size of this herniation (arrow). Note that it also extends out into the right neuroforaminal canal (curved arrow). The ability to see the association of degenerative discs with an epidural mass helps to avoid the pitfall of misdiagnosing large epidural masses as neoplasms or benign tumors. The sagittal and axial cuts through the annulus give good detail of the total anatomy of the posterior annulus. Often, what appears at first to be a mass rather than a herniation can usually be proven, on further inspection, to represent a disc herniation. This should be the most common differential diagnosis.

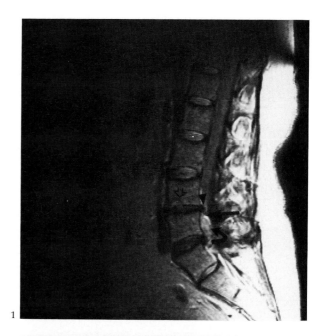

1

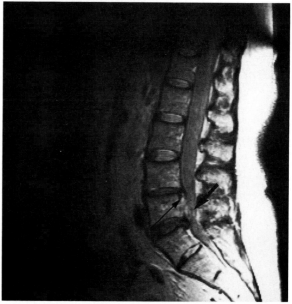

2

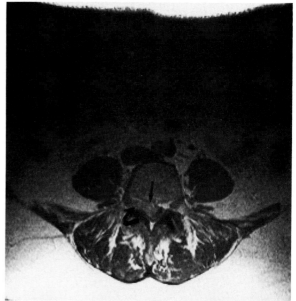

3

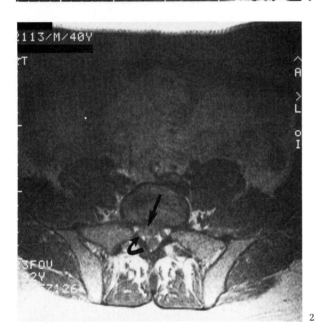

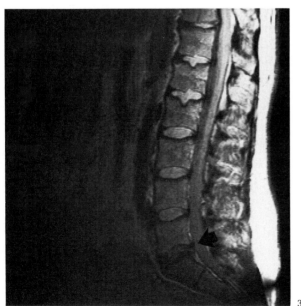

11.28 SPONTANEOUS RESORPTION OF HERNIATION AT THE L5–S1 LEVEL

Figure 1 demonstrates a disc herniation at the L5–S1 level (large arrow). Note the associated degenerative change or signal loss at the L5–S1 disc, as well as the slight retrolisthesis of L5 on S1 (long-stemmed arrow). Figure 2 demonstrates the herniation in the axial plane (large arrow). Note that the S1 root on the right has been displaced (curved arrow).

Figures 3 and 4 now MRI scans repeated approximately 8 months after the initial exam. No surgery has taken place. Note that on Figure 3 the herniation is no longer apparent (large arrow). The axial cut through this level (Figure 4) also demonstrates the decrease in the extradural mass seen earlier. Also, compare the now normal appearance of the right S1 root, which is surrounded by a normal amount of fat (curved arrow).

We can inspect the soft tissues posteriorly in the paraspinal and subcutaneous regions to ensure that no surgery has taken place. The lamina can be visualized, and laminotomy defects can be seen with MRI.

This is an interesting case. I am not totally certain of the significance of a case of this sort, but there is no history of any percutaneous discectomy, chymopapain treatment, or surgical intervention to explain this regression of a herniation. Perhaps this patient was extremely compliant with conservative rest. We will watch for more of these apparently spontaneous cures in the future.

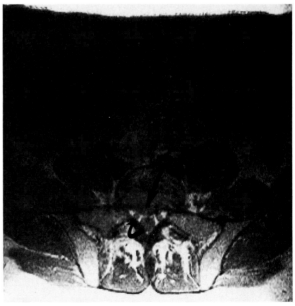

11.29 INTRASACRAL MENINGOCELE WITH SPINA BIFIDA OCCULTA

Figures 1a and 1b show the thecal canal to be expanded in the sacral region (large arrows). This is consistent with an intrasacral meningocele. Normally, these are incidental findings. On Figure 1a, the curved arrow demonstrates the normal course of the filum terminale. Figure 2 is a T2-weighted image again demonstrating that the enlargement in the sacral region and its content behave similarly to the CSF elsewhere in the spine. Figures 1a and 2 also demonstrate a congenitally small L4–5 disc space.

Figure 3 demonstrates absence of development of the lamina on the left side at the L5–S1 level. This is consistent with spina bifida occulta.

The detection of an intrasacral meningocele, with a normal position of the cord and no abnormal content within the meningocele, is usually of incidental interest. There are other congenital features here that also help to substantiate the diagnosis of intrasacral meningocele rather than that of a very large multiple Tarlov's cysts, which are perineural diverticula surrounding the roots.

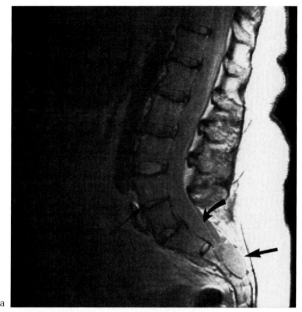

1a

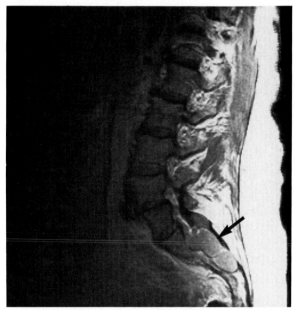

1b

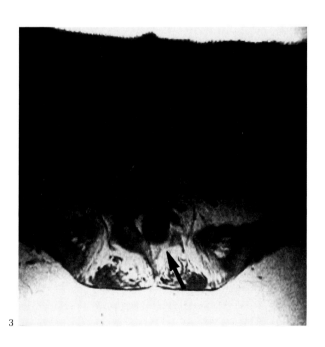

3

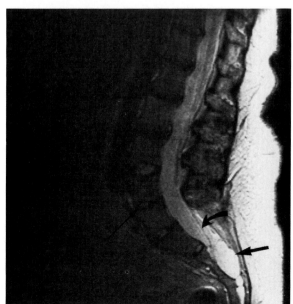

2

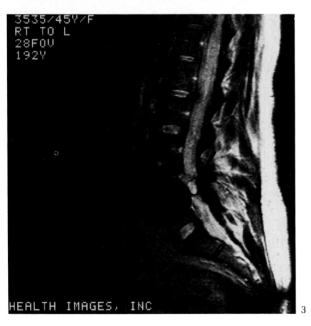

11.30 SYNOVIAL CYST ARISING FROM THE LUMBAR FACET

Figure 1 demonstrates a cyst arising from the synovium of the facet (small arrow). The large arrow indicates its continuity with the synovial lining of the joint. The joint space itself can also be visualized on MRI, and the highland cartilage surface of the facets can be seen (open arrows). Figures 2 and 3 demonstrate the T1 and T2 sagittal images, showing the fairly large size of this synovial cyst (large arrows). Note that it can create a mass effect but does not represent a herniation. The annulus is intact posteriorly at the L4–5 level, although there is some degenerative loss of signal (curved arrow).

REFERENCES

TUMORS

Vanel et al.: *Radiology* **164**:243, 1987.
Petterson et al.: *Radiology* **164**:237, 1987.
Ehman et al.: *Radiology* **166**:313, 1988.
Lee et al.: *AJR* **149**:557, 1987.
Yuh et al.: *AJR* **149**:765, 1987.
Rubenstein et al.: *AJR* **152**:685, 1989.
Dalvika et al.: *AJR* **152**:229, 1989.
Resnick: *AJR* **151**:1079, 1988.
Cohen et al.: *Radiology* **167**:477, 1988.
Abcelwahab et al.: *AJR* **149**:1207, 1987.
Cohen et al.: *AJR* **150**:1079, 1988.
Resnick: *AJR* **150**:249, 1988.
Wilson et al.: *AJR* **150**:349, 1988.
Demas et al.: *AJR* **150**:615, 1988.
Sartoris et al.: *AJR* **149**:457, 1987.
Bloem et al.: *Radiology* **169**:805, 1988.
Rosen et al.: *Radiology* **169**:799, 1988.
Siegel et al.: *Radiology* **170**:467, 1989.
Munk et al.: *AJR* **152**:547, 1989.
Sugrinura et al.: *Radiology* **165**:541, 1987.
Yogler et al.: *Radiology* **168**:679, 1988.
Kumar et al.: *Radiographics* **8**:749, 1988.
Kransdorf et al.: *JCAT* **12(4)**:612, 1988.
Bolen et al.: *JCAT* **12(4)**:681, 1988.
Dick et al.: *AJR* **151**:537, 1988.
Kaplan et al.: *Radiology* **164**:441, 1987.
Petterson et al.: *Radiology* **167**:783, 1988.
Gillespy et al.: *Radiology* **167**:765, 1988.
Tang et al.: *Radiology* **166**:205, 1988.

KNEE

Kulkarni et al.: *JCAT* **10(3)**:445, 1986.
Baurne et al.: *Mayo Clinic Proc.* **63**:482, 1988.
Haggar et al.: *AJR* **150**:1341, 1988.
Burk et al.: *AJR* **150**:331, 1988.
Hall et al.: *AJR* **150**:1107, 1988.
Goldman et al.: *AJR* **151**:1163, 1988.
Jelink et al.: *AJR* **152**:337, 1989.
Senac et al.: *AJR* **150**:873, 1988
Mitchell: *Radiology* **171**:25, 1989
Mink et al.: *Radiology* **170**:823, 1989.
Malghem et al.: *Radiology* **170**:566, 1989.
Spritzer et al.: *AJR* **150**:597, 1988.
Tyrell et al.: *Radiology* **166**:865, 1988.
Lee et al.: *Radiology* **166**:861, 1988.
Yulishet et al.: *Radiology* **165**:149, 1987.
Manco et al.: *Radiology* **163**:727, 1987.
Stoller et al.: *Radiology* **163**:731, 1987.
Mesharzadeh et al.: *Radiographics* **8**:707, 1988.
Crues et al.: *Radiology* **164**:445, 1987.

Schwinmer et al.: *Radiology* **154**:175, 1985.
Gauld et al.: *JCAT* **11(6)**:1096, 1987.
Crues et al.: *MR Clinical Sympos.* **3**:2, 1988.
Herman et al.: *Radiology* **167**:775, 1988.
Mink et al.: *Radiology* **167**:765, 1988.
Deutsch et al.: *AJR* **152**:333, 1989.

SHOULDER

Kieft et al.: *AJR* **150**:1083, 1988.
Seeger et al.: *AJR* **150**:343, 1980
Blair et al.: *Radiology* **165**:763, 1987.
Castagno et al.: *AJR* **149**:1219, 1987.
Zlatkin et al.: *AJR* **150**:151, 1988.
Mitchell et al.: *Radiology* **168**:699, 1988.
Stiles et al.: *Radiology* **168**:705, 1988.
Seeger et al.: *Radiology* **168**:695, 1988.
Evancho et al.: *AJR* **151**:751, 1988.
Kieft et al.: *Radiology* **166**:211, 1988.

WRIST

Middleton et al: *AJR* **149**:543, 1987.
Erichson et al.: *AJR* **152**:1013, 1989.
Bunnell et al.: *Radiology* **165**:527, 1987.
St. John et al.: *Radiology* **158**:119, 1986.

FOOT

Yulish et al.: *JCAT* **11(2)**:296, 1987.
Noto et al.: *Radiology* **170**:121, 1989.
Redd et al.: *Radiology* **171**:415, 1989.
Rosenberg et al.: *Radiology* **176**:489, 1988.
Kneeland et al.: *AJR* **151**:117, 1988.
Keyser et al.: *AJR* **150**:845, 1988.
Rosenberg et al.: *Radiology* **169**:229, 1988.
Huller et al.: *AJR* **151**:355, 1988.
Solomon et al.: *AJR* **145**:1192, 1986.

HIP

Rush et al.: *Radiology* **167**:473, 1988.
Johnson et al.: *Radiology* **168**:151, 1988.
Shuman et al.: *AJR* **150**:1073, 1988.
Mesgarzadeh et al.: *Radiology* **165**:775, 1987.
Turner et al.: *Radiology* **171**:135, 1989.
Pay et al.: *Radiology* **171**:147, 1989.
Glichstein: *Radiology* **169**:213, 1988.
Mackisz et al.: *Radiology* **162**:717, 1987.
Coleman et al.: *Radiology* **168**:525, 1988.
Geny et al.: *Radiology* **168**:521, 1988.
Bloem et al.: *Radiology* **167**:753, 1988.
Beltron: *Radiology* **166**:215, 1988.

TRAUMA

Berger et al.: *Radiographics* **9**:407, 1989.
Bodne et al.: *JCAT* **12(4)**:608, 1988.
Deutsch et al.: *Radiology* **170**:113, 1989.
Lee et al.: *Radiology* **169**:217, 1988.
Flechenstein et al.: *AJR* **151**:231, 1988.
Yao et al.: *Radiology* **167**:749, 1988.
Wilson et al.: *Radiology* **167**:757, 1988.
Blunenkopf et al.: *AJNR* **7**:722, 1986.

ARTIFACTS

Shellack et al.: *AJR* **151**:811, 1988.
Braun et al.: *AJNR* **7**:997, 1986.
Breger et al.: *AJNR* **9**:825, 1988.
Suojanen et al.: *JCAT* **12(2)**:349, 1988.
Curtin et al.: *AJNR* **10**:19, 1989.

INFECTION

Quinn et al.: *JCAT* **12(1)**:113, 1988.
Yuh et al.: *AJR* **152**:795, 1989.
Unger et al.: *AJR* **150**:605, 1988.
Beltran et al.: *Radiology* **164**:449, 1987.
Post et al.: *Radiology* **169**:765, 1988.
Angtusco et al.: *AJR* **149**:1249, 1987.
Sharif et al.: *Radiology* **171**:419, 1989.

CERVICAL SPINE

Mirvis et al.: *Radiology* **166**:807, 1988.
Reynolds et al.: *Radiology* **164**:215, 1987.
Teresi et al.: *Radiology* **164**:83, 1987.
Yuh et al.: *Radiology* **164**:79, 1987.
Engmann et al.: *Radiology* **166**:467, 1988.
Tarr et al.: *JCAT* **11(3)**:412, 1987.
Ehara et al.: *AJR* **151**:1175, 1988.
Bundschuh et al.: *AJR* **151**:181, 1988.
Castillo et al.: *AJR* **150**:391, 1988.
Hedbey et al.: *AJR* **150**:683, 1988.
Aisen et al.: *Radiology* **165**:159, 1987.
Lery et al.: *Radiology* **169**:773, 1988.
Post et al.: *Radiology* **169**:765, 1988.
Cyervionne et al.: *Radiology* **169**:753, 1988.
Larson et al.: *AJR* **152**:561, 1989.
Petterson et al.: *AJNR* **9**:573, 1988.
Berquist et al.: *Radiographics* **8**:667, 1988.
Karneze et al.: *AJNR* **8**:983, 1987.
Ho et al.: *Radiology* **169**:87, 1988.

Ross et al.: *JCAT* **11(6)**:955, 1987.
Czervionte et al.: *AJNR* **9**:557, 1988.
Mulls et al.: *MR Clinical Sympos.* **3**:5, 1989.
Brown et al.: *AJNR* **9**:859, 1988.
Ho et al.: *AJR* **151**:755, 1988.

THORACIC SPINE

Roosen et al.: *JCAT* **11(4)**:733, 1987.
Holtas et al.: *JCAT* **11(2)**:353, 1987.
Enymann et al.: *Radiology* **165**:635, 1987.
Smoker et al.: *AJNR* **8**:901, 1987.
Colman et al.: *JCAT* **12(3)**:423, 1988.
Ross et al.: *Radiology* **165**:511, 1987.
Dormont et al.: *AJNR* **9**:833, 1988.
Minami et al.: *Radiology* **169**:109, 1988.
Francavilla et al.: *JCAT* **11(6)**:1062, 1987.

LUMBAR SPINE

Hueftle et al.: *Radiology* **167**:817, 1988.
Heithoff: *MR Clinical Sympos.* **3**:3, 1988.
Koschoreh et al.: *Radiology* **167**:813, 1988.
Naidich et al.: *Radiology* **167**:761, 1988.
Modic et al.: *Radiology* **166**:193, 1988.
Yuh et al.: *Radiology* **169**:761, 1988.
Jinkins et al.: *AJNR* **10**:219, 1989.
Wilmink et al.: *AJNR* **10**:233, 1989.
Haughton: *Radiology* **166**:297, 1988.
Wienreb et al.: *Radiology* **170**:125, 1989.
Hesselink: *AJR* **150**:1223, 1988.
Johnson et al.: *AJR* **152**:327, 1989.
Modic et al.: *Radiology* **168**:177, 1988.
Rubin et al.: *Radiology* **166**:225, 1988.
Massanyk et al.: *AJR* **150**:1155, 1988.
Bundschuh et al.: *AJR* **150**:923, 1988.
Grenier et al.: *Radiology* **171**:197, 1989.
Frocrain et al.: *Radiology* **170**:531, 1989.
Jackson et al.: *Radiology* **170**:527, 1989.
Yuh et al.: *Radiology* **170**:523, 1989.
Grenier et al.: *Radiology* **170**:489, 1989.
Manaster et al.: *AJNR* **7**:1007, 1986.
Ho et al.: *Radiology* **168**:469, 1988.
Monajati et al.: *AJNR* **8**:893, 1987.
Ross et al.: *AJNR* **8**:885, 1987.
Cyervionke et al.: *MRI Clinical Sympos.* **4**:1, 1988.
Kaplan et al.: *Radiology* **165**:533, 1987.
Grenier et al.: *Radiology* **165**:517, 1987.
Hochhauger: *AJR* **151**:755, 1988.

Index

341